HOSPITALS IN CRISIS: A DIGITAL SOLUTION

Innovations that Save Time, Money & Lives.

by
David Veillette, FACHE

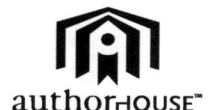

authorHOUSE™

1663 LIBERTY DRIVE, SUITE 200
BLOOMINGTON, INDIANA 47403
(800) 839-8640
WWW.AUTHORHOUSE.COM

© 2005 David Veillette, FACHE. All Rights Reserved.

No part of this book may be reproduced or transmitted in any form or by any means, electronic or mechanical, including photocopying, recording, or by any information storage or retrieval system without written permission from the copyright holder, except for the inclusion of brief quotations in a review.

First published by AuthorHouse 06/16/05

ISBN: 1-4208-5097-0 (sc)

Library of Congress Control Number: 2005903550

Printed in the United States of America
Bloomington, Indiana

This book is printed on acid-free paper.

The TIHH logo and related trade dress are trademarks of The Indiana Heart Hospital and may not be used without written permission.

Information contained in this book has been obtained by the author from sources believed to be reliable. However, because of the possibility of human or mechanical error by our sources, by the author, or by others, the author does not guarantee the accuracy, adequacy, or completeness of any information and is not responsible for any errors or omissions or the results obtained from use of such information.

The Indiana Heart Hospital is part of the Community Health Network in Indianapolis, IN. Visit their website at Hearthospital.com

Dedication

To my parents, Omer and Cecilia Veillette, who provided me the foundation of my life. Thank you for continuing to watch me and guide me from your heavenly home.

Foreword

Fleet Admiral Chester Nimitz won the war in the Pacific for America. Subsequently, he retired from active service and became Chairman of the Bulova Corporation. One day, he attended a briefing by a precocious young man; at its conclusion, the fabled five-star sidled up to the youngster and requested that their picture be taken together. When asked why, Nimitz is said to have replied, "When his vision shakes the world, I want to have been seen standing next to him at the inception."

That's me! I want to have been seen "standing next to" Dr. David Veillette when his book, *Hospitals in Crisis: A Digital Solution*, becomes the trendsetter/upsetter it will most assuredly be.

I am not an expert in David's world. I don't pretend to be. But there are some things I know. Regardless of your view about healthcare financing and the like, it's a simple fact that (1) hospitals kill and wound far too many people through inattention to tested quality-improvement methods; and (2) despite the superb disciplinary training of staff, acute-care centers have been far too reluctant to embrace anything approaching the full value offered by the new information technologies.

Enter David Veillette and The Indiana Heart Hospital. Opening on February 14, 2003, TIHH is arguably our nation's best example of what inspired, safe, technologically cutting-edge acute care can look like.

I'd love to give you some pithy quotes from David's book. But I can't. You see, I underlined *the whole darned book*. The devil is in the details, and every paragraph drips with practical and philosophical advice. I'll leave it to you to paw through the stunning fine points. I will simply say that David Veillette paints a portrait of modern, effective healthcare that is eminently doable…and a million miles from conventional practice.

TIHH is relentlessly devoted to sophisticated, thoughtful care. The new IS/IT tools that this facility has implemented have revolutionized (big word, deserved word) every aspect of the patient service process, from check-in to procedure to release and follow-up.

I am 62. My future will undoubtedly depend on the excellence (or lack thereof) of our acute-care centers. Though I live in "medically sophisticated" Boston these days, I'm frankly not optimistic. I know that extraordinary care is possible. Alas, I also know that it is not the standard, even at our "best" facilities.

Lee Scott leads Wal*Mart. Howard Schultz leads Starbucks. But if you are interested in my nominee for "best CEO," then read this book. It is not a book about "moving cheese." It is no fable…although the results are so bizarre it sometimes feels that way. This is *non-fiction*. This is a *tale of unexpected excellence…that you can learn from*. Lee Scott? Fine fellow! Howard Schultz? Great guy! But David Veillette gets my Vote as America's Best, Most Innovative and Determined CEO.

Read. Underline. Absorb. Act.

My life depends on it.

Tom Peters
Co-author of the international best-selling book,
"In Search of Excellence."
London
2005

Acknowledgements

There are so many to acknowledge for helping in the writing of this book. Without each and every one of them, this endeavor would not have been possible. Unfortunately, thanking every single great person I have met during my 30-year career is not possible. For those who I may have missed, please know that your influence and impact on my career was never underestimated.

To my wonderful wife, Jill, for all her encouragement and support. A special thanks to my children: David, Michelle, Re'Becca, Nicole, Danielle, and Aimee, who have given me the experience and wisdom of patience. You were, by far, the best training camp in how to deal with different attitudes, behaviors, and personalities. Thanks to you, this has become my strength.

I have had great mentors throughout my career. Some I have worked for and with; others I have learned from through their writings and teachings as I developed my career. Special thanks to Tom Peters, Tom Rice, Noel Tichy, Walt Disney, Jack Welch, Dave Jones, James Eastham, and Charles Bryant, M.D., whose writing, support, counsel, and advice have been critical to my development.

Thanks to my colleagues, friends, and confidants who have provided an ear to listen, support to try, challenges to improve, and friendship to encourage my often radical behaviors: Barry Hamp, Susan Holbrook-Preston, and Mary Gamache.

To the physicians of The Indiana Heart Hospital, whose openness and commitment to change made TIHH the most successful and recognized model for the hospital of the future. Without their uncompromising passion for exceptional patient care, we would not exist. My thanks to each one of you for your continued support and commitment, and to the many others involved and responsible for the success of TIHH.

To the TIHH Board, thank you for giving me this unique opportunity to put my proverbial money where my mouth was to create a new and futuristic approach to healthcare. A very special thank you to Mike Alley and Michael Venturini, M.D.

Thanks to the exceptional working managers of TIHH who continue to demonstrate and model our culture of the golden rule. Each of you recognized and embraced the changes in this new environment. To borrow the immortal words of *Star Trek*, you "boldly go where no one has gone before." Many thanks for your support and commitment. I would also like to thank the support staff we share with the Community Health Network to make the operation of TIHH a success. In addition, we could not function without the incredible dedication and talents of our administrative staff: Cheryl Williams, Cindy Benoit, and Elaine Pfenning. Thanks for keeping us all organized.

To the wonderful and insightful people from GE Healthcare who, along with TIHH leadership, recognized that healthcare needed a significant change and to that end were willing to risk their credibility and, in part, their success. Together we continue to improve the journey.

My sincere thanks and appreciation to Sheri Riley Roman, who kept me focused on writing this. I appreciate her tireless efforts in organizing, editing, and directing my thoughts into words. Kate Shoup Welsh has my gratitude for copyediting and polishing.

Most importantly, I wish to thank each and every employee of TIHH. Without your commitment to our golden rule culture and your fanaticism for customer service, our success could not occur. Each of you makes TIHH a place in which it's a pleasure to work and provide care. Thank you for what you do daily. You make me a better person—a person who loves what he does and has seen his vision become reality.

Table of Contents

Dedication v

Foreword vii

Acknowledgements ix

Introduction xiii
    Symptoms of an Ailing System xiii
    The Cure for Healthcare xiv
    Healthcare: Mission Versus Business xv
    A Call for Change xvi
    A Message of Hope xviii
    The Indiana Heart Hospital xix
    Suggestions xxi

Chapter 1
    Design 1
        Baby Boomers 2
        Suggestions 8

Chapter 2
    Fanatical Customer Service 11
        Concierge Service 12
        Room Service 14
        Golden Rule Service 15
        Suggestions 17

Chapter 3
    Physicians 21
        Partnering with Physicians for Best Results 23
        Suggestions 25

Chapter 4
    Information Technology 27
        Using IT to Generate EMRs 28
        Using IT to Improve the Work
        Environment and Quality of Care 31
        Using IT to Reduce Medical Errors 32

- Choosing Vendors 34
  Transitioning to an IT-Enabled Environment............34
  Suggestions 37

Chapter 5
Nurses and Staff...39
  A Day in the Life of a Hospital Nurse....................... 41
  TIHH's Approach 43
  Fighting Nursing-Staff Turnover.............................. 44
  A Word about Agency Nursing 45
  Support Staff..46
  Suggestions 47

Chapter 6
Insurance 53
  A Call for Change 54
  Dealing with Medicare and Medicaid 55
  Caring for the Uninsured 56
  Caring for People with Chronic Conditions 57
  A Word on Socialized Medicine.................................58
  Suggestions 58

Chapter 7
Legislation, Regulatory Bodies, and the
Specialty Hospital 61
  The Stark Laws 63
  A Key Solution: Partnering with Not-for-Profits....... 64
  Using Legislation to Improve Healthcare 64
  Regulatory Bodies 66

Final Thoughts 69

Introduction

"The one who says it cannot be done should never interrupt the one who is doing it."

—*Anonymous*

Healthcare is broken. In fact, I think it's terminally ill. Whose fault is it? Absolutely every discipline within the system can take part of the blame. That includes patients, physicians, the government, insurance and managed-care companies, vendors, and pharmaceutical companies. We've all had a hand in creating this giant, inefficient system, and now it's out of control. We need a cure, and we need it immediately.

Symptoms of an Ailing System

What are some of the problems with healthcare? The average patient has high expectations and high demands, yet wants quality care with an unlimited access to providers. Of course, they want the least expensive price. Various government entities continue to provide new and complicated ways to reduce payments and support. Regulatory bodies, like the Joint Commission on Accreditation of Healthcare Organizations (JCAHO), require countless documents and reports. These well-intentioned organizations add little benefit to healthcare but add major costs. In the pursuit of patient safety, the Federal Drug Administration (FDA) adds billions of cost to healthcare products due to its inefficient structure and endless procedures. Supplier and vendor companies provide new products and new technologies as they continue to charge exorbitant prices in the United States. Because of the significant regulatory hoops in the United States, vendors need to recoup research investment dollars here while selling the same products in other countries at one-half to one-third lower prices than in America.

As an industry, we're facing a significant loss of available healthcare workers. Nursing staffing levels are reaching an all-time low, with fewer and fewer people looking at careers in healthcare. Patient safety issues are a major concern. Hospitals and healthcare organizations are watching the bottom line deteriorate. Chief Executive Officers (CEOs) wrestle with reimbursement concerns, personnel shortages, and capacity problems. Physicians are overstressed, overworked, and feeling bled to death by insurance premiums and Health Management Organization (HMO) requirements. Physicians haven't paid attention to the writing on the wall, and they now face unprecedented attacks on their profession—not to mention their incomes. There are continuous attacks by the government and hospitals to erode away their authority and their ability to control the patient environment. Many have just looked away. I compare this to the boiling frog theory: Drop a frog in boiling water and he'll jump right out. Put a frog in cool water, gradually turn up the heat and he'll stay in the water and boil to death.

Healthcare organizations continue to operate as poorly designed, ineffective, inefficient dinosaurs. We've created environments that are not conducive to employee satisfaction, professional fulfillment, or patient comfort. Yet we continue to build healthcare organizations using the same old models, and we continue to manage them in the same old way.

The Cure for Healthcare

Fortunately, there is a way out.

We can treat and even heal our ailing system. It doesn't involve a magic pill, and it may not be easy. Are these answers all-inclusive? No. But by implementing the strategies outlined in this book, we can be on the road to recovery in a short amount of time. The strategies that we're outlining will improve the operational efficiencies, allow for better workflow and provide a better work environment. This is true for doctors and nurses. Most importantly, it improves patient care. If we continue to ignore the problems of our current system, however, we will jeopardize the healthcare of citizens of the U.S. and the world.

Healthcare: Mission Versus Business

Why does healthcare need to change? Healthcare in its entirety (that is, hospitals, doctors, insurers, suppliers, and pharmaceutical companies) is the number-one business in the world. Although many industry insiders believe that healthcare is not a business, asserting instead that healthcare is a service or a mission, I disagree—especially for hospitals. An itemized cost breakdown of the federal Gross National Product (GNP) lists healthcare costs at $1.7 trillion. This is the largest portion of the GNP. How can we afford to treat this industry as anything other than a business?

Assuming we are dealing with a business, healthcare has to be the most poorly run business in the world. The return on investment (ROI) for most hospitals is dismal. Procedures are lax. Laws that regulate the industry are confining and often at cross-purposes. Reimbursements negotiated by powerful insurers leave hospitals and doctors with barely enough money to cover costs; when companies are satisfied with a 3–5 percent profit margin, something is wrong. No other business would be satisfied with this inefficiency. Reinvestment is often impossible because the bottom line won't support it. In any other industry in the world, these conditions would prompt the immediate replacement of the Board of Directors, and the CEO would be fired. Yet in healthcare, we find this acceptable and we allow it to continue.

Many people in our profession fall back on the age-old explanation: mission. This word fits with the image of Clara Barton tenderly caring for the ill, but then she didn't have to consider documentation, liability, and insurance coverage. Healthcare workers can support the mission through the care they provide, but too often this word is used as a buffer to justify poor performance (or even non-performance) and as an excuse to avoid working to develop and implement more efficient and effective processes. Especially in not-for-profit organizations, the mission is what makes low margins acceptable. Regardless of the structure of the organization, we need to be aggressive and innovative. We need to provide better care at lower costs. We need to elevate customer satisfaction to new levels. We can no longer be content with the status quo.

A Call for Change

The fact is, entire industries have had to reinvent themselves. Telecommunications, manufacturing and financial services are just a few examples of industries that recognized the need to change or die. Yet most healthcare leaders remain closed to new ideas—often for very selfish reasons. In the old mindset, especially in not-for-profit hospitals, a CEO's stature, salary, and success are determined by bed count and by the number of employees. The CEO of an 800-bed hospital with 3–5 percent net income is considered significantly more successful and powerful than the CEO of an 80-bed facility with 10–12 percent net income. Why would he or she be interested in downsizing to find efficiencies? Why would any CEO challenge the current way of doing business if he or she would actually feel a salary penalty or suffer the loss of stature?

Besides, I've noticed that most people, CEOs included, feel that change is good—as long as that change doesn't affect them. Put another way, doing the right thing sounds good in theory. Unfortunately, however, doing the right thing often forces us to look at our own failures and shortcomings. And frankly, although healthcare has never been a well-oiled machine, up until now, it has limped along just fine—which means that painful self-examination has not been necessary. Today, however, we face perilous new challenges with higher costs, reduced reimbursements, and more sophisticated customers. The limping-along days are over. We are faced with a plethora of new problems and demands. And in response, every facet of the system is pointing fingers and placing the blame elsewhere.

To present but a few problems: Why are we still developing hospitals with semi-private rooms? Why do we defend the cold and sterile environment? Why is hospital food such a joke? We run healthcare professionals and support staff out of the very environment that needs them the most, yet pay others to perform tasks that are redundant or, in many cases, no longer beneficial to the patient or the organization. It's almost like we're determined to add discomfort and difficulties for our patients and our employees. We're inviting crisis management. It's time for an innovative approach to providing healthcare and an end to the major areas of dysfunction in most hospitals.

These are just a few of the factors that support the need for a new healthcare delivery system—a system that incorporates, supports, and leads in the areas of information technology (IT), customer service, and innovative patient and staff workflow in an environment that feels homelike and promotes healing. Courageous and innovative thinkers will look at this new environment as a major opportunity to redefine the healthcare world; others will bury their heads in the sand. Whatever their instinct, however, CEOs must address these issues head-on. Rebuild the trust with your doctors. Involve yourself with the staff. Find the time to work on legislative issues. The best CEOs will lead the charge in the aggressive and passionate changes that are desperately needed to succeed.

As you read the chapters in this book, you will notice that I have provided comments and suggested actions at the end of each one; this is so that you can implement the changes you feel warrant immediate attention, without having to read the entire book before getting started. These ideas have been successfully implemented elsewhere; use them—and any other innovative and creative approaches you can think up—as a kick-start for you and your organization. If you determine your greatest areas of need and immediately implement some of these suggestions, I am confident you will see positive results. Whatever suggestions you deem useful, I urge you to take a risk; unlearn your bad habits of the past; and embrace the new healthcare paradigm. As with many things in life, the greater the risk, the greater the reward.

A Message of Hope

Although healthcare is in dismal shape, I believe there is hope. Allow me to share a recent example. One of our partner hospitals admitted a young, pregnant woman who was in a lot of discomfort. Due to immediate access to her prior records, a very smart Emergency Room physician realized that her discomfort was not pregnancy-related. In fact, it was due to a repair of a congenital heart defect. There was a potentially fatal dissection of the aorta (a separation of the layers of wall tissue in the major artery taking blood from the heart to the body.) Within minutes, this young woman was transferred to our hospital with doctors and staff on stand-by. All the necessary data was instantly available to The Indiana Heart Hospital caregivers prior to her arrival. Anesthesia was prepared, tables were set, and surgeons were scrubbing as the patient arrived. Through extraordinary teamwork, an obstetrician and team were immediately performing a cesarean section to save the baby. Once the baby was delivered and placed in an incubator, the cardiovascular surgeons opened the mother's chest and repaired her heart. It was a near-fatal event with a happy ending. On December 16, 2004, we hosted this young mother and her beautiful baby girl to celebrate the child's first birthday. All the doctors and staff who were involved in the delivery and surgery brought presents to celebrate this exceptional Christmas present. I was proud and humbled to be a part of it. People and talent saved their lives. Technology was the enabler that made the difference between failure and success.

The Indiana Heart Hospital

The Indiana Heart Hospital (TIHH) in Indianapolis, Indiana has not just embraced the future; we're helping to define it. This revolutionary hospital, a member of the Community Health Network, opened its doors on February 14, 2003—St. Valentine's Day. This day held great marketing significance to us—a heart hospital opening on the day the world celebrates matters of the heart. We had the unique opportunity to start from scratch and do it right from the ground up. Even without that opportunity, however, the ideas and concepts from our experience can be implemented in any hospital, regardless of size or complexity.

A group of cardiologists and cardiovascular surgeons, staff, and innovative leaders were committed to developing a better environment for cardiac patients. Our vision was to be the premier provider of cardiovascular care in the Midwest. Of course, we demanded the highest level of technical expertise. Just as importantly, we wanted to create an experience and environment that resulted in the highest possible level of safety and satisfaction for the patients, their families, and their caregivers.

TIHH is an innovative, freestanding cardiac hospital—the first of its kind in the country. It's the first all-digital, paper-lite cardiac hospital. *Paper-lite* is defined as having no paper charts, no chart racks, and no medical records department. Because some government entities still require some paper documentation, we are forced to create forms, but after we achieve the paper compliance, we scan the data into our electronic charts and eliminate the paper trail.

From our architectural design to our fanaticism for customer service, TIHH is a place of wellness, diagnosis, treatment, and recovery. Every day, our exceptional people attain extraordinary results in this exemplary facility.

No stone was left unturned in the planning process. Following the groundbreaking in June 2001, the project took 20 months to complete at a cost of $65 million. Through visionary leadership, physician participation, and clinical input, the project was completed on time and under budget. Utilizing a single vendor partnership with GE Healthcare, we attained the IT integration desired by the physician partners and clinicians. In an era of rising healthcare costs, decreasing clinical resources, and concerns for safe care delivery, the IT component was vital to all parties. We knew our benchmarks of success would include customer/patient satisfaction, clinical quality benchmarks, and financial benchmarks.

Our objective was to build an environment with safety in mind. Through a collaborative effort of physicians, administrators, clinical staff, and outside partners, we set about to make our vision a reality. Several teams of various stakeholders were formed. There was staff input on every element—the design of patient rooms, equipment, documentation systems, and care-delivery models. The IT systems were implemented using a super-user concept, with each super-user being a staff member who was trained to understand, teach, and support all aspects of our IT systems. These individuals were culled from different departments and shifts to make IT support available 24/7, and were relieved of patient-care responsibilities to learn and then teach the new technology to our more than 300 staff members. Communication, in the form of team meetings, network presentations, and community forums, kept interested parties apprised of the progress and design. Focus groups of prior patients were conducted to guide us in customer expectations. A leadership newsletter, *The Pulse*, is now circulated bimonthly. An Employee Council was formed to facilitate communications within and between departments. This council is still in existence today, and makes decisions regarding dress code, employee-retention and-recognition strategies, annual celebrations, and criteria for our employee assistance fund, which is a fund that is supported and contributed to by employees for employees.

TIHH was created for the patient to have the utmost in care, diagnosis, treatment, and intervention—a concept we then took even further by looking at the physicians and staff as customers. As the CEO, my customers are the staff and doctors. If I can make their jobs easier and their day-to-day situations better, they in turn will ensure that their patients have a better experience.

Today's healthcare environment is riddled with obstacles. It's simply not conducive to providing quality care or customer satisfaction. The structures and processes in place today preclude any opportunity for real change. Since opening, however, TIHH has demonstrated significant improvements in patient safety, customer satisfaction, reduced costs, improved staffing levels, and innovative process improvements. We've taken everyone's wish list into account. Our numbers have proved that we're efficient, and TIHH has been profitable since opening day. The following chapters will look at many examples from TIHH and demonstrate that healthcare can be fixed.

Suggestions

- Invite key doctors, administrators, and a mix of staff members to discuss what each group needs in order to enhance performance. What would make their jobs better? Once these items are identified, put together an action plan to implement changes that will improve the workflow for all. Schedule a monthly meeting for this group to discuss results of the action plan. Each action needs to have a champion who guides the team to meet the objectives of the action plan.

- Use your EMS (Fire Department) to help design or improve the design of your Emergency Room services. Their input can be invaluable in evaluating your ambulance-to–Emergency Room connectivity and will enhance patient care at arrival.

- Bring your primary vendors to the design table. Often, vendors and hospitals have completely different objectives. If you're all at the same table, discussions between a hospital and its vendors can meet the hospital's needs as well as provide mutual and aligned processes, saving money down the road.

- Set up a council of employees, one from each department, either selected or elected by his or her co-workers. These individuals become the unofficial leaders of their departments. Give this council the leeway to make recommendations, handle communication, and implement changes to benefit the work environment. This will require some relinquishing of authority by CEOs and senior management. Allow the employees their say. In our experience, the council is very beneficial and, not surprisingly, has made some very intelligent decisions for our hospital.

Chapter 1

Design

"We should be taught not to wait for inspiration to start a thing. Action always generates inspiration. Inspiration seldom generates action."

—*Frank Tibolt*

At The Indiana Heart Hospital, we deal every day with patients who have heart disease or the threat of a cardiac problem. These people are nervous. Often, they are looking at their mortality head-on. Not surprisingly, they experience increased stress levels and adrenaline just by walking in the door of a healthcare facility. It makes you wonder why so many hospital environments are so cold and austere, square rooms within square buildings, boxes within boxes. Such environments only contribute to the patient's anxiety level, which can result in the need for additional pain medication, not to mention troubles with insomnia and other side effects!

We at TIHH wanted to create a different experience for our patients. Our goal in designing the hospital was to immediately reduce that stress level by providing an environment that is bright and cheery, based on the theory that the healing process can be helped by comfortable and uplifting surroundings. Specifically, the facility had to be warm and inviting. It had to be fully functional, and it had to be the best use of space that we could imagine. And no boxes within boxes for us; we at The Indiana Heart Hospital decided to think outside the box. The result? TIHH is a gorgeous facility from an aesthetic standpoint, one that truly stands out architecturally. Partnering with two firms, RTKL and BSA Life Sciences, we built the hospital of the future. Beyond that, it's a comforting and nurturing space. Most importantly, we've created a design with an improved, efficient workflow for staff and doctors.

Baby Boomers

Who did we have in mind during all this planning and discussion? It's very simple: the baby boom generation. This generation of people, born between 1943 and 1964, has affected our society in every way imaginable, and as boomers become older, you'll want to hold on to your seatbelts! We're all in for an interesting ride. Here are just a few tidbits about this amazing group of people:

- There are nearly 77 million baby boomer Americans, and only 44 million Gen-Xers in line behind them.

- Baby boomers are set to be the next retirement generation, yet they are also most likely to be in a sandwich situation—simultaneously caring for aging parents and for children still at home.

- Baby boomers don't consider themselves "senior citizens" and they don't want anyone else to either.

- Although boomers are aware of the need to be proactive in maintaining good health, many are not doing so. In 2002, 38 percent of younger boomers (aged 35 to 44) and 31 percent of older boomers (aged 45 to 54) were current users of some sort of tobacco. A significant portion of the boomer population is overweight and many are obese. Most do not get the recommended level of exercise. These are all factors that can contribute to cardiac disease.

Source: the-info-shop.com by Global Information, Inc.

HOSPITALS IN CRISIS: A DIGITAL SOLUTION

This generation single handedly has, and will continue to have for many years to come, the greatest impact on healthcare. From health insurance to attitudes about health issues, they are the driving force. For this reason, the design of our facility factored in the lifestyle of the average baby boomer, in conjunction with elements to promote healthy living. Here are but a few design decisions that we made after analyzing our core group of patients, the baby boomers:

- Aging baby boomers are going to require cardiac care. Some consulting firms try to tell the public that preventive healthcare and the overall wellness effort will kick in and decrease these numbers. I don't see that. In fact, our country needs to be prepared for the onslaught of cardiac patients. We're in the worst shape we've ever been.

- Every patient room in our hospital is private. In addition, every room in TIHH is ICU-capable. We move the nursing staff to the patients—not the patients to the nursing staff. In a typical scenario at a traditional hospital, a cardiac patient changes location about three times during his or her stay, even if the stay is only four days. The patient goes from the surgical ICU to a step-down unit to another unit before being released. With every location change comes a necessary paper trail—everything from admissions and discharges to medications and medical orders must follow. And with every change, there's the possibility for unnecessary errors and trauma thanks to lost orders, paper mix-ups, and medical complications. For instance, suppose you have a patient with bad veins for whom you have finally managed to insert a stable IV. When you move the patient to a different unit because he or she is doing better, you run the risk of losing

- the IV; if this happens, the physician may well have to order an invasive procedure for the IV, which means you've just added to the length of stay, not to mention the patient's discomfort and possible complications. You're also amplifying the risk of infection. In addition, frequent movement is stressful to patients and their families. This is not a scenario that's conducive for caring for patients. Making every room ICU-capable can make an amazing difference in a patient's length of stay.

- If you ask nurses why they entered their chosen profession, most will say to make a difference and to care for people. Yet hospitals have effectively removed nurses from the bedside for 44 percent of their work schedule. One of the ways TIHH has addressed this issue is by eliminating the nursing station. There is no central unit where nurses must go for charts, instructions, or anything else. By supplying a computer in every room and decentralizing the nurses, we've put them back at the sides of their patients, which is where nurses want to be.

To support this decentralized model, we designed each floor in TIHH to resemble a propeller. In the center of the propeller is a greeting desk with room for minor secretarial support. Radiating from this center area on each floor are three pods; the nurses in each pod are completely self-sufficient. Each pod has eight private rooms, and is stocked with its own set of medications, supplies, linens, and nutrition areas. In addition, every room in every pod is identically stocked. The furniture and equipment are in the same place, as are the medications and supplies—right down to the linens in the drawers. This design, a direct result of input from the staff, ensures that everyone who works in a pod has everything they need to be successful at their job right at their fingertips.

HOSPITALS IN CRISIS: A DIGITAL SOLUTION

Although part of why this design works so efficiently is because it is completely enabled and supported by our information technology, our design can also be implemented and significantly improve staff flow in a paper world. This design has had a tremendous impact on the lives of our nurses, and more importantly, on the lives of our patients.

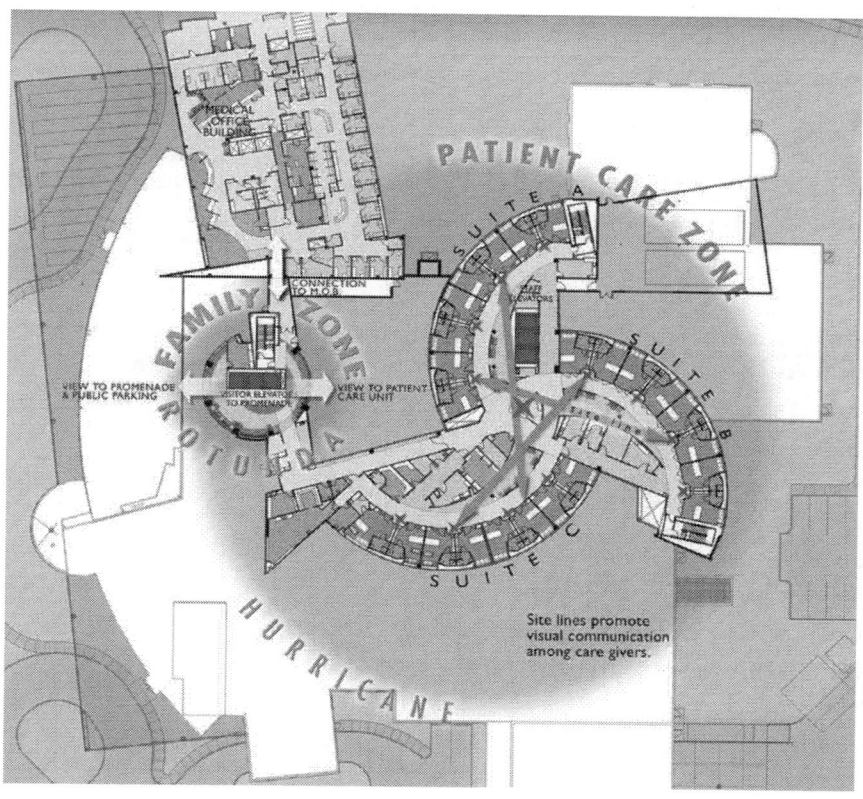

Site lines promote visual communication among care givers.

David Veillette, FACHE

In a typical healthcare environment, nurses often need to float from one unit to another. For example, one unit may be extraordinarily busy and call on a nurse from another unit to help. Problems arise when the nurse who has been called is not familiar with the unit or when the patient care needed is not his or her expertise—for example, a cardiac nurse assisting in the neurology unit. This situation is frustrating for everyone involved, and wastes significant time. One nurse is trying to help, but must overcome a learning curve in order to do so. Another nurse, who needs assistance, spends valuable time teaching, directing, and supervising. This can't be the best scenario for the patient!

At TIHH, each nurse stays within his or her own pod. Making a habit of transferring nurses from one pod to another would defeat the purpose of our design. As a rule, we operate with one nurse to four patients (this ratio does not include the nursing support staff). But instead of focusing on nursing ratios, we use the patients' actual and perceived needs to dictate the level of nursing care. If two nurses are needed for one patient, then we make that happen. If one nurse can handle eight patients, then we make that happen. Nonetheless, we have designed our pods so that if you are required to use nursing ratios instead of acuity (illness) to determine your staffing needs, the worst-case scenario is one nurse to eight low-acuity patients. Very rarely, situations arise that require us to shift nurses from one pod to another; in our scenario, we have kept this to an absolute minimum.

HOSPITALS IN CRISIS: A DIGITAL SOLUTION

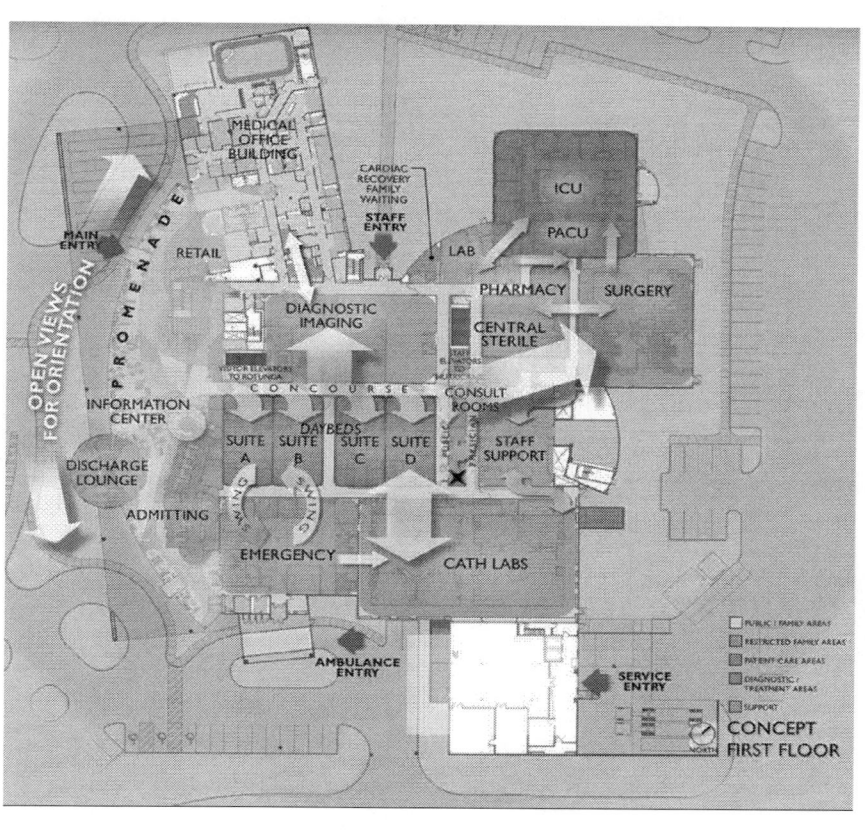

Suggestions

- Consider a new design. Make sure to involve the staff to get their ideas for improved flow. Listen to the suggestions and, most importantly, implement them.

- If you believe that bad habits (such as smoking) contribute to diseases, make a statement against those habits with your policies and facility design. For example, even though we understand, and often cater to, the desires of the baby boomer generation, we created a non-smoking campus. There are no "smoking areas" for staff or patients anywhere on the premises. It can be unpopular, but we believe our role as a heart hospital—and yours as a healthcare provider—requires a non-smoking facility.

- Many experts agree that within the next 10–15 years, the only patients in hospitals will be those who are critically ill and require Intensive Care Unit rooms. Why build a plethora of general patient rooms that cannot support ICU patients? TIHH built all ICU-capable rooms with this belief in mind. The 400 (or 500 or 600+) bed hospitals will be unused and tragically wasted facilities in a few years. Don't think in the short-term, and don't waste your energy and money on ineffective facilities.

- As you look at your design plans, challenge the status quo of every area. Find a better way to decentralize the pharmacy through the use of medication units on the floor. By allowing your nurses more control over medication delivery, you require fewer pharmacists and pharmaceutical technicians. Challenge the need for every nursing station.

- Create areas to de-stress. Design comfortable break rooms away from the patients. Include outdoor space in the overall design. Garden space and walking trails give staff and patients a soothing environment to decompress and heal.

Chapter 2

Fanatical Customer Service

"Excellence can be attained if you risk more than others think safe, care more than others think wise, dream more than others think is practical, expect more than others think is possible."

—*Anonymous*

Regardless of the beauty of the building and the incredible IT system that enables our staff, quality care still comes down to people dealing with people. That's why we at TIHH are fanatics about customer service.

Fanaticism means "excessive enthusiasm." I love that definition. These days, there's a lot of lip service about providing customer service. Pick up an annual report or look at the marketing materials for just about any company, and they all tout their commitment to customer-service. But very few of us can point to an organization that, day in and day out, really seems enthusiastic—and certainly not *excessively* so—about the topic. Indeed, most of us have countless horror stories of bad service: searching for someone to help us, dealing with rude clerks, suffering automated machines when we just want to speak to a person, the list goes on.

Think about your most recent frustrating experience with customer service. You probably don't have to think too long. Now, imagine yourself in that frame of mind with the added stress of having a heart attack or a cardiac scare. Even routine medical tests can send adrenaline levels sky high. This is a situation where customer service is needed most, and generally found the least.

Before I go too far here, let me define *customer*: Every person who walks through our door is our customer, but first and foremost, our customer is the patient. Why do I insist that this is so? Because in healthcare, patients are treated differently from customers. After all, because patients need service because of illness or injury, most hospitals believe the patient needs the hospital more than the hospital needs the patient—hence, poor service. But when you think about *customers* rather than *patients*, you expect a different level of service. We want to do everything possible to make the experience at TIHH as comfortable as possible. That includes the family. If I do my job and the families feel engaged with the staff and doctors, that confidence transfers to the patient. It reinforces the quality of care and relieves patient stress.

As the CEO, I also view the administrators, doctors, and staff as customers—*my* customers. If I'm going to expect extraordinary customer service from them, I had better set a benchmark by providing it to them. We look at everything they do, every day, to try to find ways of making their jobs easier. My job is to take the pebbles out of their shoes. Every solution I can devise enables them to do their job more effectively.

Concierge Service

When most hospitals talk about customer relations, it's just a buzzword. Usually, it means that they have one, maybe two people whose sole purpose is to appease angry patients or families by offering them a free meal or some other minor perk. At TIHH, we created an entire concierge department—12 people—dedicated to guest relations. As concierges, their entire job is to make life better and easier for our customers: patients, staff, doctors, and families.

Most people associate concierge service with hotels. In that capacity, the concierge will make your dinner reservations, store your luggage, and get your theater tickets. So will our concierge service. They will do almost anything that needs to be done. Whether you're a patient who needs an errand run or a doctor who needs a bank deposit made, it doesn't matter. We'll handle it. This amazing group of people coordinates a multitude of tasks every day. They will get your tires changed; they'll take your car for a lube job; they'll drop off your laundry and pick up your concert tickets; they'll arrange your child's birthday party or anything else that will make your life better and your stay more comfortable.

Because working in a hospital can be a high-stress environment, we have massage therapists from a local massage school come in once a week. Car washes are available in the parking lot every Friday afternoon. There's a Starbucks Coffee shop in our lobby. Drycleaning pick-up and delivery is also available. During the busy holiday season, staff can drop off lists of presents they need, and the concierge staff will do the shopping and even wrap the presents for the staff to pick up and put under the tree. By including the staff in this service, we've reinforced the value we place on them. No one needs to coordinate errands in the middle of the day; our concierge staff will take care of it. This allows our doctors and staff to focus on our patients, knowing that these minor tasks are in good hands.

Last year, a patient of ours experienced a massive heart attack on April 13th. After he was stabilized, he was scheduled for surgery on April 15th. He notified the concierge service that all his income-tax information was spread out on his dining room table. The concierge went to the man's home, picked up the information, helped him complete the necessary documents, and had it all to the post office before the April 15th deadline. Just taking a worry off someone's mind can make a world of difference in the quality of his or her care, not to mention the patient's overall hospital experience.

David Veillette, FACHE

Room Service

In the traditional hospital, a tray is delivered to every patient, even though some patients may be out of their rooms due to surgery or other procedures, or they may be sleeping or recovering from a procedure. An hour later, the absent or sleeping patient's untouched tray is retrieved and the food is tossed. A few hours later, when the patient is awake and hungry, the best the nurse can offer is some juice and crackers.

At TIHH, you can forget tray delivery—we offer room service 24-hours a day, seven days a week, at no extra charge. Patients and staff alike can call the kitchen as often as they like to receive their food made to order (unless the on-duty nutritionist deems that the ordered food conflicts with doctors' orders for a patient). Think about the patient who's admitted at 8:00 p.m. Maybe he's been in the Emergency Room for a couple of hours, and now he's hungry. In the traditional hospital, he has to hope the kitchen can come up with a sandwich or something. In our environment, he just picks up the phone to order a complete hot meal.

Believe it or not, we're actually saving significant amounts of money with this service. Why? Because this model ensures that the food we provide is not wasted. And although hospital food has been a running joke since, well, forever, one of the highest ratings we receive on patient surveys is for our food. That's because in addition to being available any time, day or night, it's actually *edible*. At TIHH, we have executive chefs whose sole responsibility is to ensure that the food is excellent. We're a heart hospital, so we offer high-quality, heart-healthy food. We're sodium and calorie-conscious. At the same time, we are realistic about the likelihood of changing the eating habits of anyone in a two- to three-day period. If a patient requests a specific food and it does not conflict with the physician's orders, we will accommodate the request. As a result, our patients and staff are all eating the same high-quality, great-tasting food.

Golden Rule Service

I believe in the golden rule: Do unto others as you would have them do unto you. For this reason, TIHH is a "golden rule" environment and culture. This explains why all our rooms are private and include a foldout sofa and a large recliner chair, allowing families to stay with their loved one. On many occasions, I have received comments from families who were very pleased to be able to stay. One woman expressed surprise that our staff even provided clean towels and supplies for a shower after a long night. Another family member couldn't believe the staff provided fresh linens for the foldout sofa each morning.

Customer service goes beyond amenities like towels and sheets, however. For true change, we knew we had to blow up the old-fashioned systems and reinvent our processes. We asked, "What can we do to make this a better place to work and care for people?" This is not an easy question to answer. As a rule, healthcare organizations don't ask how to improve workflow or problem-solve for staff—or if they do, perhaps by issuing an "employee survey," very few actually attempt to change the environment. Sure, they act like they care, putting teams together to discuss the surveys and develop action plans, but in most cases the plans have no meat and no real hope of addressing employees' needs. Alternatively, many organizations depend on national customer-satisfaction tools and boilerplate consultant solutions without resolving any issues.

Worse, it's the rule, rather than the exception, that the CEOs and administrators of hospitals don't even know what's going on in their own organization. These people rarely leave their offices, and absorb all information from whatever reports happen to land on their desks. I won't operate that way, and I won't support an organization like that. How can you know what is going on with your staff, your doctors, and your patients if your most vital information is coming to you second and third hand? For this reason, I schedule 90 minutes every day for a walkabout. I walk through the hospital and I talk to everyone whose path I cross. I learn more from the walkabout than any report or presentation that comes my way. In addition to helping me determine what's really happening on the floor, I find that my walkabouts please the staff. They are happy to know that if they have an issue, I will be around, and they can discuss it with me.

Some of the simplest problems can be fixed during a walkabout. On one occasion, two nurses caught me on my walkabout and told me that if their unit could just have a blanket warmer, their patients would be happier, and they could provide better care. It just so happened that on a walkabout the day before, I noticed two blanket warmers in our ER. I asked the ER Director whether the ER really needed two warmers, and before the end of the day, a warmer "mysteriously" arrived in the nursing unit. A simple problem—and because of the walkabout, I knew where and how to fix it. Why let a problem fester into a major complaint? Part of the solution is being visible and being available.

Not convinced? Consider this story: Not too long ago, a technician mentioned to me that the lead apron rack in the radiology unit was inconveniently located. If the rack could be right outside the appropriate door, the physician or technician could grab the garment on the way in. Instead of waiting days for maintenance request forms to make their rounds, I used a screwdriver to fulfill the technician's request in a matter of minutes. In addition to resolving the problem, this simple act demonstrated that someone was listening. After all, don't we all want to feel like our opinion is important? I've told everyone at TIHH, "Be careful of what you ask for because I will probably give it to you."

In addition to my daily walkabouts, I make it a point to be present at odd hours. It may be easier to work a 9–5 schedule, but I don't do that because this hospital is open 24/7. It's not uncommon for me to come in at 2:00 in the morning and cook omelets for the night shift and for families of patients in the Emergency Room. To support our night staff, we also have night hours for the gift shop and the Starbucks™ Coffee shop. I schedule monthly morning meetings, called "Donuts with Dave," and afternoon meetings, called "Cookies with Dave." I let every person, regardless of their shift or stature, know that I am available to hear their stories and work toward a solution.

At TIHH, we listen, change, try again, change, improve, change again, and implement new processes quickly and without concern for failure. After all, how can you provide customer service without asking the doctors, staff, patients, and families what they want and need? It's impossible. Never, I repeat *never*, assume you know what they want. Ask them.

Suggestions

- All concierge and food services are free, with no tipping permitted. Among our many offerings, we have valet parking and greeters at the front entrance.

- We require every department manager to greet and valet park cars for one hour a week between the hours of 11:00 am and 2:00 pm so the guest-relations staff can enjoy lunch and to allow a face-to-face dialogue between our managers and our patients.

- Every family waiting in the lobby for a loved one receives a beeper. This allows the family to go to the restaurant or simply to walk around without fear of missing any updates or physician conferences. It also eliminates the need to call out patient names—a clear violation of HIPAA guidelines.

- A family liaison is responsible for checking on patients during procedures and keeping the family informed at least once every 30 minutes.

- The family liaison guides families back to one of the four consultation rooms to visit with doctors after procedures.

- We hold two monthly meetings with our volunteers, who we believe are critically important. In our meetings, volunteers discuss issues, make suggestions, and update activities. We always provide cookies, coffee, and juice. Managers rotate participation in the meetings, during which they explain their department's role and ask for input to improve their area.

- We provide a thorough Preferred Provider List to patients, families, staff, and physicians. Our concierge staff visits all the local hotels, restaurants, and other services in the area to solicit discounts for our customers. Our list is extensive and runs the gamut from inexpensive to moderate. We've even negotiated free nights at local hotels for patient families who cannot afford the lodging expense.

- Allow a little frivolity. We've made a sticker available that allows staff to wear nice jeans on Fridays. The proceeds of the sticker sales go to the Employee Assistance Fund. To boost morale, we hold drawings for staff for prizes—makeovers provided by a local beauty college, tickets to a ballgame, and so on.

- No aimless wandering is necessary. We've made it our policy to ensure that everyone is accompanied by an escort or volunteer to get to their proper destination. We've all been in the frustrating situation where we're told to turn left here, pass two hallways, and then take a quick left—the result being we end up walking in circles trying to find our destination. Families are often distracted, frightened, or tired, and this guidance is immeasurable in the overall experience.

- Consider using doctor and patient concierges. In our environment, the patient is greeted upon arrival and the concierge makes sure everything is taken care of. Every doctor has a personal concierge to ensure that phone calls are returned in a timely manner, to provide meeting and procedure reminders, and to run any necessary errands.

- Avail yourself of nearby high schools and colleges to develop a pipeline for recruitment. Recently, we partnered with a local high-school marketing class. We sponsored one of two teams to develop, market, and analyze results of selling rubber bracelets. These types of partnerships benefit the school and the community. Also, by interacting with students in this manner, we fostered an awareness of healthcare and all of its different variables as a viable career choice for these students.

- At Christmas, ask carolers from area schools perform for staff and visitors.

- Look at attitude above attributes. We all want to hire the most qualified people, but I know plenty of technically competent people who are incapable of holding a pleasant conversation with colleagues or patients. The basic skill base is important, but a positive, can-do attitude is critical. Customer-service skills are of monumental importance. I believe that people who are hateful, unfriendly, and unapproachable are simply lazy. It takes work, and a lot of it, to be outgoing, friendly, and considerate. This should be the norm. As you go through the hiring process, pay attention to attitude. You'll see people who are qualified but lazy. You'll also see people who are gregarious and willing to work on the skills required. You make the choice.

Chapter 3

Physicians

"One of the most sublime experiences we can ever have is to wake up feeling healthy after we have been sick."

—*Rabbi Harold Kushner*

Allow me to be brutally honest. We can talk all day about return-on-investments, nursing shortages, architectural design, and much more. But the bottom line for any hospital is its physicians. Never underestimate the value and importance of placing quality physicians on your team. They are the key to your success.

Today's physicians face unique challenges. Although they are continually portrayed as rich and omnipotent, the reality is quite different. According to the Workforce Analysis Branch of the Bureau of Health Professionals, here are just a few of the statistics that affect physicians right now:

- Assuming healthcare consumption patterns and physician productivity remains constant over time, our aging population will increase demand for physicians per thousand population from 2.8 in 2000 to 3.1 in 2020.

- In 2000, physicians spent an estimated 32 percent of patient-care hours providing services to people 65 and older. If current usage patterns continue, this percentage could increase to 39 percent by 2020.

- The aging of the health workforce raises concerns that many health professionals will retire at about the same time that demand for their services is rising.

- The rise in healthcare expenditures associated with the rapid increase in the elderly population will likely place additional pressures on the Medicaid and Medicare programs, as well as private insurers, to control healthcare costs.

- The aging population could result in rising average patient acuity, which could in turn require higher nurse and physician staffing levels.

- Demand for healthcare services by minorities is increasing as minorities grow as a percentage of the population. Minorities are underrepresented in the physician and nurse workforce relative to their proportion of the total population.

Here at TIHH, we took a long, hard look at the physicians' role and how their lives could be made more productive and rewarding. One key finding was that doctors are no different from anyone else; they are as frustrated by inefficiencies as nurses, patients, and administrators. And it's no wonder! Most hospital physicians want to start their day by seeing or possibly discharging patients before they start rounds and other procedures. Instead, in a traditional hospital setting, many times the doctor arrives on the unit to find that a patient's chart is not available or, even worse, that the nurses are in a change-of-shift meeting, where they are reviewing all the charts in the unit. When the necessary chart is finally located, doctors can experience yet more frustration thanks to missing lab reports, a lack of updates from consulting physicians, or the absence of other relevant data. In a paper system, these problems can result from something as simple as a misfiled piece of paper.

Without the documentation he needs, the physician moves on to other patients, where, often, he hits the same brick wall. He does the best he can to maneuver through the bureaucracy, eventually leaving the unit to handle office patients, surgeries, or other procedures. (Keep in mind that there may still be a patient waiting to be discharged, a person who could have gone home had the necessary information been accessible.) In order to complete his duties, the doctor will need to make *another* trip to the unit—not to mention field countless phone calls in the interim from frustrated patients and family members—in order to review the patient's records, assuming those records are available.

These inefficiencies are rampant, and result in endless hours being added to a physician's day. Worse, every lost piece of data adds to a patient's length of stay, which means that the hospital also pays the price. The bottom line? The current healthcare environment is not designed to provide quality care to the patient, and is not capable of supporting the physicians and staff. This situation can—and *must*—be improved.

Partnering with Physicians for Best Results

When speaking at an organization or conference to CEOs and administrators, I often ask how many attendees are both MDs *and* senior leaders of their hospital or healthcare organization. Inevitably, very few hands are raised. Indeed, in most hospital systems, administrators think they, not physicians, own the revenue stream. Case in point: A few years ago, the CEO of a not-for-profit organization I once worked for actually said, and I quote, "Doctors need our hospitals more than we need them. Patients come to our hospital because of us, not the doctor." Even more frightening, he *believed* it.

As you might have guessed, I believe the exact opposite. The only person who can admit a patient to a hospital is a doctor; that means doctors are the people who control the revenue stream. Indeed, physicians can do more to reduce costs, control expenses, improve quality, improve outcomes, and boost volumes than anyone else in the organization. Despite this, administrations routinely carve physicians out of the decision-making process, keeping all financial data close to the vest. Many administrators perpetuate this mighty power struggle—which in turn perpetuates mistrust between doctors and administrators. Not asking doctors and staff for their input creates a totally dysfunctional work environment, provoking them to believe that hospitals do not care about them or their opinions. Ultimately, this hurts everyone.

Our setup at TIHH is different. Because we believe that doctors are excellent business people when given the necessary information, our Board of Directors is 60-percent physician controlled. In addition, they have a minor interest in the ownership of the hospital. The stake is hardly enough to retire on, but it does give physicians a significant voice in how our business is run, as well as in how their patients are cared for. Smart CEOs recognize the need to partner with physicians, even without a financial investment.

In our system, as the CEO, I manage the budget, but the physicians have tremendous input. If they want to spend money on something, I outline the return on investment for them. If they believe a particular purchase is necessary even if it doesn't show a return, that's fine by me. I've told them many times they can spend every dime we make, if it means patient care is improved. We all are in this together, and the quality of care outweighs cost considerations.

A perfect example is equipment purchases. A physician may attend a conference and preview the latest and greatest widget. In the old system, the machine/widget/gadget might be purchased, after much debate with the administrators, for hundreds of thousands of dollars, only to sit in the back room collecting dust because the training or supplies are too expensive. In our operation, however, we look at all the costs associated with the investment. Then, if the physicians still want it, we buy it. If it's the right thing to do for our customer, we do it. Hopefully, we can make money to cover it, but if not, so be it. Interestingly, in our model, physicians have consistently demonstrated that they make the right business decisions when given the appropriate information.

As another example of how partnering with physicians can improve the bottom line, consider the fact that as a doctor organization, you have enormous power to negotiate with suppliers. Vendors negotiate prices based on their percentage of business. If your physicians can agree to work with a single vendor, you can negotiate with that vendor to receive the best deals on products. When viewed in this light, it becomes all the more apparent that refusing to partner with your physicians is foolish and shortsighted. Our physicians are our champions. They use the system and they make it work. We have the track record to prove it.

In today's environment, doctors have to work three times as hard to make half the money they made five years ago. If increased efficiency enables a doctor can see five more patients or perform two more procedures a day, that means he or she has made more money. If there's anything you can do to make their lives better, why wouldn't they buy off on that? Just show them the benefits.

Suggestions

- Meet quarterly with your physicians. Discuss and seek input on financials, strategic plans, and customer surveys.

- Be prepared (at least in the first few meetings) for challenges and plenty of suggestions. Take quick action on these suggestions. Demonstrate your willingness to try new avenues and adapt to change. Talk through the challenges and don't be afraid to ask for help. Stop assuming that you know all the answers. You don't. Together, your team will be stronger.

- Set up a technology committee primarily made up of physicians, one from each specialty area. Give this committee the authority to commit funds or services as they deem necessary. Assign one administrator and one physician to champion any new technology, with the administrator providing returns on investment, volumes, staff issues, and so on; and the physician outlining why the technology is a medical necessity. These committees should also go back to each existing service, product, supply, and procedure to evaluate the need for modification or elimination of current practices.

- Set up a physician-driven and -controlled information technology committee. Ask this group to champion the adoption of, the implementation rate for, and success measures for converting to an IT healthcare world. Without physician commitment and the necessary ground-floor involvement in the use of information technology, no healthcare organization will move forward.

- Set up a physician-controlled steering committee for any and all service lines. CEOs: It's time to give up the control.

Chapter 4

Information Technology

"I don't fear computers. I fear the lack of them."

—*Isaac Asimov*

Most of us can't get through the day without the Internet, our cell phones, or email. Yet, those of us who are baby boomers are dinosaurs when it comes to technology. The generations at our heels are not just accustomed to the high-tech world, they *expect* it. Indeed, the children and young adults of today were exposed to a keyboard at about the same time they were learning to drink from a cup. These are our future leaders.

Although technology has radically changed our world, *Fortune Magazine* reported in 2003 that more than 90 percent of the estimated 30 billion health transactions conducted each year are handled by phone, fax, or mail. I suspect that statistic is still true. Compared to companies in other industries, healthcare companies spend a miniscule amount on information technology. Although that trend is shifting, we're still playing catch-up.

At The Indiana Heart Hospital, we have taken a different approach: We embrace technology. Indeed, it's was our view from the very beginning that information technology (IT) would be our enabler. As the first fully digital specialty hospital, we had some basic IT requirements:

- Driving everything to an electronic medical record (EMR)—including computerized physician order entry (CPOE,) dose charting, and all multidisciplinary documents—was critical. As an input tool, computers were a necessity. By choosing this course, we eliminated the need for a medical records department. We have no paper charts, we have no chart files, and we've saved a significant amount of money because of that.

- We had to improve the work environment for our staff and doctors, and IT allowed us to give them what they needed. By extension, this has improved quality of care.

- We had to address the medical errors and related issues facing healthcare today.

Using IT to Generate EMRs

Patients see a multitude of people during treatment—doctors, nurses, nutritionists, pharmacists, rehabilitation specialists...the list goes on—and all of these people need access to information about their patients. In a paper system, there's only one chart, which means that if one person has it, nobody else can see it. In the environment we've created, however, in which caregivers enter patient information into computers, 20 people can access the exact same record, or EMR, at the exact same time. We've created a facility with no runaround. The quality of care is improved because everyone has the information they need, whenever they need it.

This capability is especially critical when you consider the fact that cardiac care is often an ongoing process, not a one-time procedure. In a paper environment, records for a patient who was treated several months ago would likely be filed. But in an emergency situation, in which every second counts, the attending physician needs to know exactly what happened to a patient on a previous admission. Did the patient have a balloon angioplasty? A heart stent? If a physician has to wait for a paper chart to be found in the archives or on microfiche, the patient will probably be discharged, possibly to the morgue, before that information is unearthed. That's critically unfair to the physician and the patient. In our system, the patient's entire medical record with TIHH is available with the click of one entry field. Simply select which admission you need to see, and you have immediate access to reports, X-ray results, lab data, and even heart catheterization films. Any records received from outside organizations are scanned into the patient's TIHH electronic medical record. Immediate decisions can be made for the appropriate care of the patient.

Computerized physician order entry (CPOE) is the key to this model. It puts the control of information at the doctor's fingertips, wherever he or she may be. They can make better decisions quickly, and at the same time make fewer errors. In fact, if you're a heart patient in our facility, your doctor can review your history and issue instructions before he's even left his or her house to meet you at the hospital. We also have a cardiologist on site 24-hours a day, seven days a week, who has immediate access to EMRs. And because nurses no longer need to chase each patient's chart in order to provide care, they can now spend 80 percent of their time at the patient's bedside. Unlike traditional hospitals, which expect nurses to work a complete eight-hour shift and also make sure each patient's chart is up to date before leaving, which inevitably leads to outrageous overtime costs, TIHH nurses end each shift on time, knowing each patient's record is as it should be.

To facilitate this, TIHH, a 100-bed facility, has roughly 450 computers. With that kind of computer-to-bed ratio, you're practically tripping over a keyboard before you even have a chance to look for a pen and paper! Why? Because we recognized that for our digital system to work, we couldn't have doctors or staff jotting down patient care instructions or notes about prescriptions. Our belief was, and remains, that if you install too few computers, the physicians and staff will revert to their old paper-and-pen ways. If the equipment that doctors and staff need isn't readily available, all your attempts at efficiencies will be lost. Do not—I repeat, do *not*—attempt to save money by believing you can operate an IT hospital with only a few computers. This is critical.

In addition to making patient information accessible to anyone who needs it, using EMRs has resulted in a dramatic reduction in the use of everyday office supplies—paper, copiers, printers, fax machines, and all the other entrapments. Indeed, we save about $1 million each year on these supplies because our records, including physician order entries, MD documentation, dose charting, and other documentation, are all computerized. A recent study conducted by HIMSS for Lanier Worldwide noted that an estimated 60 pieces of paper are generated for every hospital patient visit; not so with us.

In addition, we enjoy substantial cost savings thanks to our elimination of the need for a medical records department. Consider this: In a facility our size, about 1,700 square feet of the hospital would ordinarily be dedicated to medical records. At a cost ranging from $190 to $250 per square foot, that adds up to $340,000! Add to that the human-resources costs of running a medical-records department. A facility our size would normally have three or four people managing the paper files, but we have none. Zero. There's no paper to search for or to file. Moreover, a recently conducted Six Sigma study demonstrated that we save about $2,700 per bed, per year, simply because our nurses use computer monitors to capture patient information instead of writing vital statistics down on paper and later transferring that information to a patient chart. In addition to saving money, the system enables us to avoid documentation mistakes.

Of course, like all aspects of our facility, our IT system was not designed in a vacuum. We gathered input from everyone who would use the system to design it, and we continually update it to make it better. For example, a physician might mention a change in the way the system handles a particular task that could save 20 seconds per patient. If the physician performs that task hundreds of times each day, the time savings can really mount!

To eliminate redundancy, we determined which types of information crossed multiple fields, and made sure it only needed to be entered once. At the same time, we designed the system to permit us to interact with other entities in the medical community who still use paper-based systems, and to ensure compliance with government standards. This process traditionally involves a continual paper chase. At TIHH, however, all the necessary information is gathered on the computer system before being printed out. Indeed, we have 100-percent compliance on most of the mandatory data because our computer system won't allow required fields to be bypassed by the physician or staff member who is entering patient information.

Using IT to Improve the Work Environment and Quality of Care

Chapter 3, "Physicians," discussed how frustrating it is for a physician who comes into a paper-based workplace first thing in the morning to check on his or her patients, and discharge those who are ready to return home. Faced with missing charts, disappearing lab reports, and the absence of other relevant data, the doctor is forced to put off this important task until later in the day, which translates to longer stays for patients, longer workdays for doctors, and increased costs for hospitals. At TIHH, however, doctors and nurses have all the patient information they need, right at their fingertips. Charts are updated with the click of a mouse, lab results are entered as soon as they are available, and information from consulting physicians is on hand. If a physician wants to check a chart for any reason, he or she can do that anywhere—including from home or from his or her office. This setup saves the hospital money, saves the physician time and money, and saves the patient time, money, and frustration. Through our IT system, we've not just improved operations; we've improved quality and outcomes.

David Veillette, FACHE

With regard to quality of care, TIHH meets and exceeds standards of efficiencies in the cardiac care world, as well as minimums set by the National Registry of Myocardial Infarction, with which all hospitals will have to comply in the near future. Here are but a few examples of ways in which TIHH shatters industry standards:

- Per the National Registry of Myocardial Infarction, a cardiac patient must be administered an EKG within 10 minutes of crossing the threshold into the Emergency Room. Last year, TIHH averaged 3.2 minutes from door to EKG, and it's less than that now.

- The National Registry of Myocardial Infarction asserts that patients requiring catheterization, a balloon angioplasty, or a stent should have the necessary procedure administered within 90 minutes of entering the ER. At TIHH, we average less than 50 minutes.

- In most parts of the country, the average length of stay for cardiac patients averages 4.5–4.75 days. Our average is 3.3 days.

Where would you rather be in a heart emergency? You want to be in the facility that moves quickly. Every minute you save is critical muscle saved. That's why, at the end of the day, I'll measure our quality of care against any other organization. We get our patients out of here more quickly because we don't waste time backtracking, creating redundancies, and looking for information we should already have.

Using IT to Reduce Medical Errors

The Institute of Medicine's 1999 report, "To Err is Human: Building a Safer Health System," estimated that 44,000 to 98,000 people die annually as a result of medical errors in an in-patient setting. These deaths are due to the wrong drug, the wrong dosage, allergic reactions, or a multitude of other situations. Not surprisingly, medical errors such as these result in increased costs for hospitals, estimated at $4,685 per patient, due primarily to increased hospital stays for patients—4.6 days on average. If a patient who is the victim of a medical error—or that patient's family, in the event the error proves fatal—decides to sue, hospitals can expect to pay $660,000, which is a rough estimate of the median compensation for a major award. That's only if the suit is settled out of court. Otherwise, the figure is much higher.

Having our clinical documentation online has reduced medical errors in several ways. For one, handwriting legibility is no longer an issue. In our environment, physicians use computers to enter the order of care or medication, including dosage and instructions. It's clean and clear, easy to read and understand. Perhaps more importantly, having our clinical documentation digitized helps us to avoid errors related to the administration of drugs. Potential problems, such as drug allergies or adverse drug interactions, are immediately flagged by the computer. The doctor can override the pop-up notification, but if he or she does, our system provides an audit trail that shows when and why the notification was overwritten. As a result, everyone involved with the care of that patient is apprised of the situation, and the physician doesn't make an accidental error that could've been prevented. In addition, when it comes time for a nurse to deliver the medication to the patient, he or she must first run the bar code wand over the patient's identification, over the medications, and finally over his or her own nurse's badge. Doing so enables the computer to verify that the nurse is administering the right medication for the right patient, again reducing the chances for a medical error.

Of course, we're not perfect. Anytime you have human interaction, there's potential for error. We still have the occasional instance of a caregiver misreading an order or a physician transposing letters as he or she enters a prescription. But we've made tremendous strides, and errors such as these are usually caught. The end result? We've seen an 80 percent reduction in medical errors—which has resulted in a significant savings.

Choosing Vendors

The more desires our committee outlined, the more certain we were that we wanted to work with one company that had the greatest breadth of—and best class of—products to serve our needs. At the same time, we needed a partner willing to integrate any non-partner product into the mix. We also needed someone to work with us on ongoing development strategies. We knew we would not be satisfied with a vendor who plugged in its products and disappeared. This would be a journey for the long term, and we needed a company who was willing to commit!

After many meetings, proposals, and discussions with several companies that could meet our needs—imaging, power plant, information technology, monitoring, non-invasive testing, physician office information technology, financing options, and most importantly, support and service—our decision became obvious: GE Healthcare. Our experience and results to date prove that we made the right decision. I highly recommend the exhaustive research beforehand. We have total comfort and commitment with our choice and we have the results to prove that we made the right decision.

Transitioning to an IT-Enabled Environment

We at TIHH are a digital facility, and everyone who works here must operate accordingly. In order to enjoy increased efficiency, we can't allow anyone—staff or doctors—to work around the system; sometimes, we've had to be rather hard-nosed about it. For example, a physician can't write a note or issue verbal instructions for a nurse and ask him or her to input it in the system. Not surprisingly, this has, on occasion been met with some resistance. After all, we're creatures of habit. Nobody likes to have to learn new procedures when they're comfortable with the old ones. But if you show your physicians and staff how they can save time, money, energy, and frustration by buying into your system, you'll undoubtedly get their attention! Here are some tactics we used to make the transition work:

- Gather a core group of committed physician leaders to act as champions of the system.
- Exhaustively prepare prior to "going live" on the system.
- Couple comprehensive training with realistic expectations. For example, our admitting doctors spent 8–16 hours training up front, and they continue to train as we redesign the system to incorporate their suggested upgrades.
- Provide excellent on-site support during and after the roll-out. At TIHH, we've tapped several *super-users*, who have been trained to know the system inside and out. They're available at any time on any unit. Indeed, some of our physicians have even become super-users; their excitement is contagious.
- Insist on the absolute minimization of paper or verbal alternatives.

Some additional thoughts:

- Expect an extensive process with all participants to accommodate changes, minimize overlap, and reduce surprises.

- Expect to invest significant time in building the content, looking especially at common orders, pathways, alerts, and many other fields,
- Consider going "live" for the physicians last. They have the least time to spare.
- A minimum number of training hours must be required.
- Supplement with Web-based refresher information and updates.

Here's what we found: There will be some initial awkwardness. There will be some inevitable miscommunications. You must be diligent about mitigating risk by careful auditing of the system.

Medical Records	
➢ Paper, Chart, Rack, Storage, etc.	$1,000,000
➢ Space	$ 340,000
➢ FTE (↓3.5)	$ 72,800
Charting	
➢ Nursing Time Saved	$ 151,200
➢ Triage Time Saved	$ 11,947
Staffing	
➢ Agency	$ 696,729
➢ Turnover	$ 230,000
➢ 25% Reduction	$ 1,410,573
Total Savings	$ 3,913,249

In our short history at TIHH, we have embraced technology as a tool to solve many of the problems that complicate the workings of every hospital and healthcare system. As a result, hundreds of executives, physicians, and administrators have toured our hospital in an effort to uncover the secret of our success. Yet as I guide these guests through our facility, I am continually astonished by their willingness to continue doing things the same old way. Sure, change is scary, but how can you afford not to implement it? Think of the costs involved in recruiting, retention, staff turnover, training, staff satisfaction, physician satisfaction, medical errors, paper costs, printing costs, building space to house medical records, staff to manage the records...the list goes on and on. TIHH was indeed fortunate to have the opportunity to start with a clean sheet of paper to design, construct, and implement this new hospital. However, any organization, whether existing or new, can accomplish the same results. Some may take more time than others, but the question is not "if," but "when?"

Suggestions

- Your IT partnership is pivotal. We spent many hours in internal discussions outlining what this partnership needed to look like and accomplish before ever putting out the request for proposals.

- Think broadly and for the long-term. You must make absolutely certain that any further purchases for your organization can be fully integrated into your system. No products, equipment, or services can be standalone. It completely defeats the purpose. You will find this very difficult to accomplish without a single, primary vendor. In choosing your vendor relationship(s), I suggest extreme caution. You should require proof and written guarantees that your vendors will integrate with other partners, at your discretion.

- If you're struggling with the best first step for IT integration, I suggest starting with a basic electronic medical record (EMR). The nursing staff is generally the largest part of the healthcare organization and thus will provide the greatest impact with the use of EMRs. As a byproduct, physicians will have to use portions of the EMR to recover patient data from nursing notes. This initial training by physicians will make it easier for them to move into other IT areas, such as computerized physician order entry (CPOE), dose charting, and MD documentation.

- Be committed for the long haul. Do your research and make thoughtful and thoroughly considered decisions. With the right partner, you can handle the obstacles and stay the course for long-term success.

Chapter 5

Nurses and Staff

"We shall be remembered more for...our kindness than for our accomplishment, our generosity than for our riches, our service than for our successes."

—*Anonymous*

These days, you hear a constant refrain bemoaning nursing staff turnover and the lack of available, qualified people to fill empty positions. Consider these points, supplied by nursesource.

- Unlike other nursing shortages, what we're facing now isn't about sheer numbers. It's about having nurses with the necessary specialties, skills, and experience.

- The Bureau of Labor Statistics reports that jobs for Registered Nurses (RNs) will grow 23 percent by 2008. That's faster than the average for all other occupations.

- About half the RN workforce will reach retirement age in the next 15 years.

- The average age of new RN graduates is 31. They enter the profession at an older age and work fewer years than nurses traditionally have.

Additionally, according to the U.S. Department of Labor, one in five RNs works part-time. The same organization also notes that "employment in hospitals, the largest sector, is expected to grow more slowly than in other healthcare sectors while the intensity of nursing care is likely to increase, requiring more nurses per patient." We also face a shortage of nursing faculty. Students are being turned away from nursing schools because of over-capacity.

The fact is, however, there is no shortage of nursing professionals in this country. Rather, what we have is a lack of nursing professionals who choose to work in hospitals. Why would they? As long as healthcare organizations continue to operate in the same old environment, with redundancies and inefficiencies, with paper records, without computerized physician order entry (CPOE), and with poorly designed workflow and design units, nurses are going to continue to flee. Under the current system, we run nurses out of hospitals into the open arms of pharmaceutical companies, medical insurance companies, and doctors' offices.

Think about it: When you work for a doctor's office, pharmaceutical company, or another company in the healthcare field, the hours are pretty standard—usually Monday through Friday, 8 am to 5 pm. The base pay is comparable to hospital pay, and there may be a bonus for productivity. In addition, nursing professionals often find other perks outside the hospital environment, such as expanded healthcare benefits, childcare facilities or reimbursement, fitness centers, and other enticements.

Don't take my word for it! According to the American Health Association Trendwatch (June 2001), "Hospital employees are willing to leave for lower paying, less pressured workplaces. All together, the number of registered nurses working in hospitals went up between 1988 and 2000, yet the proportion dropped from 68 to 59 percent. A recent study found that only 51 percent of hospital employees intend to stay for several years."

A Day in the Life of a Hospital Nurse

Nursing can be an enormously rewarding profession—but it can also be one of the most frustrating. In fact, according to a recent VHA survey, one of the major problems for hospital nurses is that they are away from the patients' bedside 44 percent of the time. Instead, their time is spent chasing documents, looking for charts, tracking down doctors, and retrieving lab reports. Most nurses chose their profession for two reasons: They want to care for patients and make a difference. But how can do either when they seldom see the patient more than once during an eight-hour shift?

Let's examine a typical day for a traditional hospital nurse. He or she generally starts a shift by reviewing patient charts, which are *supposed* to be located in a central nursing station, usually found in the middle of the unit, far removed from the majority of the rooms in the ward. When the doctors arrive on the unit, the nurses gather the necessary charts for the physicians to check on their patients. Sometimes all the paperwork is where it is supposed to be, but unfortunately, this is the exception, not the rule. As many nurses will tell you, it's not unusual for lab results or other important information to be missing from the chart. Maybe they haven't been sent from the lab, maybe they've been misfiled, maybe they're incomplete—the reason doesn't matter. The bottom line is that the information needed is not available. And so, as the nurse embarks on a valiant search for the necessary information, the physician moves on to the next patient. Meanwhile, who do you think bears the brunt of the physicians' justifiable frustration? The nursing staff.

As another example, consider the problems that nurses face when attempting to read a physician's order of care. A few years ago, the Institute of Medicine estimated that 98,000 people are affected adversely every year as a result of medication errors, and poor handwriting was one of the listed causes. In addition to having to interpret chicken-scratch penmanship, nurses are forced to figure out which drugs to administer—

no small task when you consider that the names of many drugs are very similar, with only one or two varying letters to distinguish them. If the nursing staff is unable to read an order, the physician must be tracked down for clarification. This costs time, money, and sometimes even lives. In a paper-driven organization, this scenario is played out multiple times daily. The doctors are doing their jobs, the nurses are doing their jobs, yet everyone is frustrated! And on top of day-to-day patient care, government-regulated documentation is an added (and often unnecessary) stress.

This trend has not gone unnoticed. According to *Health Care's Human Crisis: The American Nursing Shortage*, the key problem is that we've taken an already stressful occupation and made it more difficult. "The burden of care on nurses has increased, yet work-saving technologies have not been implemented. At the same time, new regulations and documentation requirements take nurses away from patient care. These work environment issues create formidable recruitment and retention challenges."

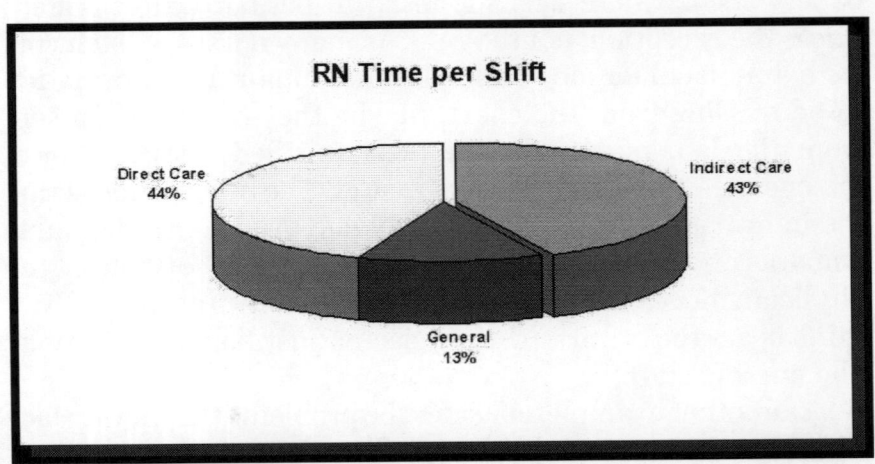

TIHH's Approach

At TIHH, we attacked the problems facing nurses by breaking the mold and redesigning the processes. To try to do everything the old way would only add to the inefficiencies. If we were going to make our nurses' jobs more fulfilling and meaningful, our first step was to ask what they needed, what would make their job easier, what we could do to help. Here were some of the responses:

- Nurses wanted more time with the patient, so we moved the nursing stations and placed both at the bedside.

- Nurses wanted a voice in the design of the hospital, so we made them part of the design team. Nurses from every department worked with administration, doctors, and designers to create rooms and units that offered maximum efficiency.

- Nurses wanted better areas to de-stress, so we placed the break rooms well away from the patient rooms and created comfortable, warm environments with couches, recliners, televisions, and other amenities. We also created a rooftop garden area, allowing staff to enjoy the outdoors during the work day.

- Nurses wanted a say in how the units were manned and operated, so we created self-directed teams on each unit.

- Nurses wanted to work with managers who embraced a positive environment, so we hired only top-notch professionals who exhibited the right attitude and who embraced our culture of fanatical customer service.

As a result of our efforts, we've seen an amazing increase in the hours of productive work. Instead of chasing charts and clarifying orders, our nurses are actually nursing the patients. The side benefits are also astounding. As but one example, consider patient falls. In the traditional hospital environment, where patients rarely see their nurses, some may try to get out of bed unassisted, which can result in a fall ranging from minor to tragic. At TIHH, however, because our nurses spend so much more time at their patients' bedside, we've seen a drastic decrease in these types of falls. The number of incidents has been cut in half, and we're well on our way to meeting our goal of zero.

To further improve the lot of our nurses, our Chief Nurse Executive (CNE) has been known to join me on walkabout; this has given us an opportunity to address many human-resource issues—things like tuition reimbursement, differential pay issues, and overtime guidelines and policies. During these walkabouts, we've also received some great suggestions from our nurses for recruitment and retention. These walkabouts do wonders for nursing-staff morale. One newly hired nurse mentioned that in 10 years of employment at another facility in town, she had never met or even *seen* the CEO. Yet, in just two visits to TIHH, she not only saw my CNE and me twice, but we both stopped to greet and welcome her. It's not rocket science—so why aren't you doing it?

Fighting Nursing-Staff Turnover

Remember the 1989 movie, *Field of Dreams*, starring Kevin Costner? There was a great line in that movie: "If you build it, they will come." Although the movie was talking about baseball, the same is true for qualified nurses and staff. At TIHH, we built a facility designed to improve the lot of nurses, doctors, patients, and family alike—and as a result, they have come.

While the news is filled with stories of the nationwide nursing "shortage," we at TIHH have a waiting list of nurses who want to work for us. And once a nurse has been hired at TIHH, he or she typically doesn't want to leave. In our first year of operation, our turnover rate was less than 10 percent; currently, we're looking at about 6 percent. Compare this to the national average of 14 percent for medical surgical nurses and 20–22 percent for cardiac nurses.

This has greatly improved our bottom line. On average, replacing a cardiac nurse costs about $55,000. That doesn't include the nurse's salary; it's just how much you spend to get a new person hired and up to speed in your facility. For a medical surgical nurse, the cost is about $46,000. If you employ 400 nurses and you lose 20 percent of them each year, it doesn't take long to figure out that you're losing millions of dollars in turnover costs. At TIHH, we enjoyed a $203,000 return on investment from the national average during our first year of operation.

In addition to saving money, improving turnover rates can in turn improve the quality of patient care. This is especially so with repeat patients. Instead of dealing a revolving door of staff, these patients derive comfort from seeing a familiar face. And because the average age of our nursing staff is 38 years old, in contrast to the national average of 44–45 years old, our nurses will likely be on the job longer, resulting in more continuity for both patients and physicians.

A Word about Agency Nursing

For most hospitals, agency nursing—that is, using an agency to fill in when you don't have a sufficient staff—is a huge cost. You pay a premium for this service. Not only does using agency nursing set you back financially, it's a disaster for morale. Think about it: You're paying an agency nurse $40–50 an hour and your own on-staff nurses are making $25–30 an hour. It's no wonder that your staff suddenly hates you! You're asking them to work side-by-side with someone who is less effective, yet gets paid more.

Before we opened TIHH, our hospital network used agency nurse services for cardiac care. Since we've opened our doors, however, we haven't spent a dime on agency nursing. Philosophically, I think it's too demoralizing to our staff. Besides, if you ask nurses, they'll tell you they'd rather work short-staffed with a lot of dedicated people than have to contend with nurses who aren't familiar with our system. Decisions like this have made a big difference at TIHH; our nursing staff satisfaction is 80 percent compared to a 35 percent national average.

Support Staff

Just as you should never underplay the importance of your nursing staff, you should never underestimate the importance of your support staff. Every member of your staff is equally important to the success of your hospital.

Many of the issues that nurses face also affect allied health personnel. In particular, many of the professional areas, such as respiratory, radiology, pharmacy, technicians, and other support staff, experience similar recruitment and retention issues; many of these workers are constantly under recruitment attack from other hospitals and industries. For this reason, all the services we provide to the nursing staff are also provided to the rest of the hospital staff; these services go a long way toward making TIHH a great place to work.

In addition to these professionals, we at TIHH greatly value those workers who man the so-called "lower-end" positions—food-service and environmental-service personnel. Indeed, at TIHH, we believe these individuals are some of our most important staff members. The work they do is critically important; just consider what happens on your units when beds are not cleaned quickly enough! Patients in the Emergency Room or various procedure rooms are kept waiting. Indeed, the environmental staff can single-handedly cause an organization to go on divert—a disastrous occurrence for a hospital that is required by law to treat any patient that enters. Obviously, these staff members play a critical role in the day-to-day lives of our organization. As such, you must take good care of them!

Because food-service and environmental-service personnel have constant contact with patients and families, whether they're cleaning rooms or delivering room-service meals, they are often the first staff members to become aware of a problem that a patient or family is experiencing. Indeed, these staff members are faced with questions from patients and families hundreds of times each day—usually the same question asked repeatedly during the course of a shift. It is critical for these staff members to remember to answer the question in same positive, upbeat, and caring manner as the first time it was asked. For this reason, we've made it a point to provide these individuals with additional, specialized training, much like the Walt Disney Company does for its "Custodial Hosts."

The bottom line? Your staff, especially your support staff, be they pharmacists, radiologists, or food-service personnel, are critical to any hospital's success. By using technology to create a new way of dealing with paperwork and regulations, we have significantly improved their work environment, and allowed them to focus on their jobs: providing unparalleled service to our staff and patients. Our extremely low turnover is evidence of our success.

Suggestions

- In the best interest of your staff, the CEO or senior leaders need to be seen on the floor and in the units, open, and available to talk. There is no easier way to make your staff feel important than to plant yourself in their work environment. Every once in a while is not enough; your presence must be constant. At first, you might meet some resistance from suspicious staff members, but eventually, you will see them open up, share concerns, and provide suggestions. They will also notice if you go out of town and have not been around.

- Be prepared in your walkabouts to answer some tough questions. You may not have every answer on the tip of your tongue, but you can resolve issues and explain why and how certain decisions are made. If someone asks you a question you can't answer, tell that person you'll find out—and then do it. Also, take responsibility for tough decisions and explain why the decided course of action was required. If you can't as the CEO, then perhaps the wrong decision was made.

- Each of us must put pressure on insurers to help compensate for smoking-cessation programs. Once an individual has successfully completed such a program, he or she should be reimbursed 100 percent for the cost of the program.

- Create a mandatory screening program for your staff. At TIHH, we have five screening elements:
  - Body Mass Index (including weight and height)
  - Cholesterol
  - Glucose
  - Blood Pressure
  - Smoking Verification

- For each area passed, the employee receives $3 off his or her bi-weekly insurance premiums; as it turns out, potentially saving $15 every other week is a great motivator! Eventually, the screening will be mandatory, and any area not passed will require a certain percentage of improvement on a quarterly basis in order for the employee to retain his or her employer-provided healthcare benefits.

- Hold a monthly book review with managers to discuss books on leadership skills. Each manager can take a chapter and lead the others in a debriefing and discussion session. In addition to leadership development, the staff discussions often lead to creative and productive solutions.

- Create a rooftop garden for nurses to eat and relax during breaks. In addition, furnish nursing unit break rooms with easy chairs, CD players with headphones, quiet areas for de-stressing, TV areas, and a small kitchen.

- Design training modules for all employees, and tie the completion of these training modules to increases in pay. For example, at TIHH, in order to earn merit increases, employees must complete at least two modules per year.

- Eliminate agency nursing. Agency nursing breeds contempt, and the whole process is self-perpetuating. As a rule, you pay agency nurses a premium above the current wages of your nursing staff. Then you overstress your staff and make them work side-by-side with someone making more money, with no emotional investment in the institution. There's no commitment; there's no obligation. The person on your staff decides to quit and work for an agency service at higher pay. You hire them back (through the agency) and you pay the agency costs. Instead, take the dollars saved by eschewing the use of agency nurses and reinvest them in better work environments. With more participation for employees and higher wages and/or better benefits, it will not take long for healthcare providers to see that agency breeding won't be supported at your hospital. You will be out of the agency circle and you will have a more dedicated staff. Since opening TIHH, we have had zero usage of agency nurse services. Prior to our opening, our partner company paid over $700,000 in 2002 for agency nurses in cardiovascular services. Think of what you could be saving and reinvesting in your staff. Bite the bullet.

- Meet with your housekeeping staff on a monthly basis to reinforce their importance to the organization and to underscore the message that they are part of the team.

- Instead of having all housekeepers be part of a central group, consider having a housekeeper for each unit and/or area of your organization who reports to the manager of that unit and who is engaged as a team member. You will also need to maintain a small group of housekeepers for the general care of common areas.

- Create multidisciplinary teams that include nurses and all other professionals and nonprofessionals alike. Encourage these teams to address room-turnover issues, medication-restocking and -delivery issues, respiratory missed treatment issues, and so on. Make sure that the housekeepers are involved so they can report the obstacles they encounter in turning over rooms, and make sure that their comments are considered and addressed. Have the team listen—really listen—to the comments that food-service and housekeeping staff overhear daily. This provides an opportunity for the others on the team to hear what patients and families are saying from someone who is non-threatening.

- The CEO, senior leaders, and managers need to meet with all support staff in different venues and with different professional responsibilities to get a broad perspective of the organization's growth and improvement opportunities.

- Obesity is a lifestyle factor that contributes to heart disease. As a patient, how much credibility do you give your nurse or caregiver if he or she is obese? Isn't that the "pot calling the kettle black?" We hired an obesity specialist to start programs for our staff and patients to address this primary cause of heart disease and other disorders. Discover ways you can create policies that contribute to the overall health and well being of your staff, as well as provide a model for your patients. Now that obesity has been classified as a disease, which Medicare and insurers will reimburse, get started and get reimbursed for successful programs that reduce obesity for your staff and your patients.

- At TIHH, we provide a fitness center with 24-hour-a-day card access for employees. We also employ a diet specialist to teach classes to both the staff and the public on obesity.

Chapter 6

Insurance

> *"A hospital bed is a parked taxi with the meter running."*
>
> —*Groucho Marx*

American newspapers and magazines routinely document the disgraceful behavior of organizations that provide health insurance to people in this country. These companies pay outrageous salaries and bonuses to executives while forcing healthcare organizations and doctors to accept continued reductions in reimbursement. The result? These insurance companies boast record profit levels of 15, 20, and even 40 percent, while doctors and hospitals generate only a 4–5 profit— every penny of which is needed for reinvestment just to keep up with demand. Meanwhile, because "medical plan premiums have risen 60 percent since 2000, despite a general drop in administrative costs" (source: *CIO Insight*, November 2004)—a number that far outpaces the 7 percent increase in the nation's total healthcare bill, which itself is more than double the inflation rate—more than 40 million Americans go without any health insurance at all. The scariest thing of all is, although physicians and healthcare providers know how to treat many chronic diseases and illnesses, no one is willing to pay them to do so.

It's no wonder that the November 2004 issue of *CIO Insight* called healthcare the poster child for dysfunctional business models. The magazine noted that insurers are interested in trimming the costs charged by providers, "but only by using their vast numbers of customers as leverage to dole out less money, rather than by installing technology to create the collaborative networks that could improve communications between payers and hospitals." Even if an insurance company does invest in IT, it rarely does so in order to improve care for their customers. According to the *CIO Insight* report, "Aetna, the No. three medical insurer, recently completed a $20 million overhaul of its data systems—the goal being to identify physicians who are prescribing procedures and drugs too liberally, among other things."

It's time to face the fact that managed care has not worked. Moreover, it will not work in the future because it involves diametrically opposing goals. Healthcare organizations and physicians are challenged to provide quality care, to make a small profit that must be reinvested for the future, and to provide charity as part of its mission. Yet managed care insurers are charged with running a business with shareholders who demand returns on their investment. Insurers and healthcare providers end up butting heads instead of trying to find a sound solution for everyone—an approach that ends up lowering the quality of healthcare.

A Call for Change

The design and implementation of a digital hospital can allow phenomenal efficiencies, significantly reduce costs, and improve quality on all sides of the equation. Even in the face of poor reimbursements, digitalization and improved workflow designs can help hospitals operate efficiently enough to run more effectively and to generate a reasonable profit. But insurers must be forced to examine their part of the mix.

First and foremost, insurers must limit the demands they make on hospitals and doctors. It is simply not acceptable to continue to ask healthcare providers to limit their profits to a measly 4–5 percent so that the CEOs of insurance companies can enjoy $40 million bonuses and other perks.

Beyond that, insurers should be forced to invest some of those enormous profits in wellness programs. The fact is, we treat the sick instead of helping the healthy remain healthy, when we must do both. If we had truly useful programs to encourage wellness, fitness, and early health screenings, we would provide a better quality of life not just for our patients, but for the country in general. But because these programs don't boost their bottom line, insurance companies have no interest in paying for them.

Insurers are not entirely to blame for the state of healthcare today. As I've said, everyone involved in healthcare has contributed to its disrepair. Insurers are, however, in a unique position to start moving healthcare in a more positive direction. They have the ability and the profitability to make significant strides in turning this disaster around. The astronomical profits need to be reinvested in wellness programs and in the support of doctors and hospitals. A continuation of the current system will only lead to the demise of health insurance. If business decisions continue to be made at the expense of patients, enrollees, hospitals, and physicians, the system will not survive.

Dealing with Medicare and Medicaid

Medicare and Medicaid are sources of additional insurance nightmares in part because the government reimburses hospitals for services performed by paying a relative value for medical procedures. Every illness has a relative value. For example, a heart surgery might have a relative value of 6.5, with the hospital receiving $1,000 per unit, or a total of $6,500 for the procedure. Minor procedures receive lower values, while more complex procedures receive higher reimbursements. A side effect of this system is that it places specialty and physician-owned hospitals under attack by not-for-profit hospital systems, who claim that specialty hospitals are skimming off the high profit margin business and leaving the high acuity, bad debt, and charity work for the not-for-profit healthcare systems. Creating a new payment system could help.

I suggest that Medicare equalize the payment for all diseases. Instead of paying higher values for diagnostic related groups (DRGs) in Cardiology and Orthopedics, why not issue equal payments for all based on the true acuity (seriousness of illness) of the patient? Equalization would eradicate concerns about skimming services. The problem that is then created is that digital and specialty hospitals would remain profitable because of the efficiencies gained through IT. But because the not-for-profit hospitals know their operations are inefficient, they still could not generate a reasonable profit, so this approach would cause them to lose *more* money which is why they have no interest in this solution.

Caring for the Uninsured

In a statement to the House Energy and Commerce Subcommittee on Oversight and Investigations, it was reported that in an effort to recoup costs, hospitals routinely charge uninsured people up to four times as much as insured people. As indigent patients are unable to pay, insured patients must pay more; meanwhile, the uninsured are subjected to debt collectors. When you consider that an estimated 43 million Americans have no health insurance, and that countless others have inadequate coverage, it becomes clear that millions of us are but one Emergency Room visit—and certainly one catastrophic illness—away from personal bankruptcy. Where are the high-profit insurers in this scenario?

I do not believe there are quick fixes or easy solutions for these very complex problems. But all involved parties—hospitals, doctors, insurers, and the government—*could* come together to develop a comprehensive plan for human wellness and basic coverage for the uninsured. It cannot be the responsibility of one entity of healthcare; all of us need to address the problems and resolve these issues. It must be done in such a way that the patients and their needs are put first, and the profits of shareholders and hospitals are considered second. Unfortunately, this can never happen as long as hospitals and doctors with a mission to serve are standing diametrically opposed to insurers whose goal is profits—not to mention the government, which proceeds with a tunnel-vision, cost-reduction outlook. We've been living in this mindset for far too long.

Caring for People with Chronic Conditions

According to the Center for Studying Health System Change (*Issue Brief #88*, Sept. 2004), about 57 million working-age Americans (18–64 years old) live with chronic health conditions such as diabetes, asthma, and others. These conditions hit low-income populations particularly hard. The idea of medical bills that they cannot afford often causes people to forgo or delay treatment or to fail to get proper medication due to cost concerns. According to the report, "problems are especially acute for the uninsured. Forty-two percent went without care, 65 percent delayed care and 71 percent did not fill a prescription because of cost concerns." Even those *with* insurance grapple with this problem; According to the same report 10 percent of insured patients with chronic health conditions have gone without care, 30 percent have delayed care, and 43 percent have failed to fill a prescription due to cost concerns.

Again, there is no easy answer for these problems. Should pharmaceutical companies be forced to provide drugs for the uninsured at no or very low cost? If the insurers could provide basic healthcare needs and cover more preventive care with their huge profits, perhaps hospitals would be not have to make up for the losses of the uninsured and underinsured—therefore becoming even more effective in delivering healthcare. Whatever the solution, each entity is going to have to begin putting the needs of patients above all other considerations.

David Veillette, FACHE

A Word on Socialized Medicine

One potential solution to the problems facing healthcare today is socialized medicine. In a nutshell, under a socialized system, private insurers disappear, and all healthcare costs are paid by a government healthcare fund. In theory, this practice provides care to every citizen. In practice, however, its pitfalls are great and plentiful. For this reason, I don't know anyone in the healthcare industry—myself included—who believes that socialized medicine is the answer. But as Congress continues to feel the public pressure to examine these unchecked profits of insurers, some reaction is certain. If insurers want to avoid the implementation of socialized medicine—a move that would obviously run them out of business—they'd be wise to take heed.

Suggestions

- Insurers need to invest in IT to improve, enhance, and expedite the claims process. This IT approach should involve an expedited pre-certification process. The time wasted by healthcare organizations to get authorization to treat patients is unnecessary and does not add to quality or efficiencies for the insurers or the hospitals.

- Insurers need to encourage wellness by covering the costs of providing education by hospitals. If insurers do not want to pay hospitals to provide such programs, then they should provide these programs themselves, or at the very least provide wellness credits to patients. If insurers believe in wellness, then they should be required to put their money where their mouth is.

- Insurers and legislators need to seriously examine and change the bonuses, incentives, and salaries of insurance executives. These enormous profits are made off the backs of the general population—common men and women, many of whom are just trying to make ends meet.

- Insurers need to consider using their high profits to offset medical- and nursing-school costs—for example, implementing and paying seed money and education and training costs. There is a need to reinvest in increasing the pipeline of doctors and nurses to work in the hospital for the future. Demand it.

Chapter 7

Legislation, Regulatory Bodies, and the Specialty Hospital

> *"The marvel of all history is the patience with which men and women submit to burdens unnecessarily laid upon them by governments."*
>
> —William H. Borah

As I indicated at the beginning of this book, the failure of healthcare has enough blame to go around. Everyone is at fault. Yet, aggressive lobbying efforts by groups like the American Hospital Association and many of the larger not-for-profit hospital systems would have you believe that specialty hospitals, especially those with physician ownership, are single-handedly causing the collapse of the not-for-profit healthcare system. They contend that physician-owned specialty hospitals are skimming all the profitable service lines, such as cardiology, orthopedics, and ambulatory surgical services, while leaving the poorer reimbursement lines, charity cases, and bad debt cases for the not-for-profits.

Not surprisingly, I disagree. In fact, it's my view that what these groups are *really* demonstrating is the frailty of our healthcare system—that a movement so small in scope, the specialty-hospital movement, could have such a significant perceived impact.

David Veillette, FACHE

Here's a dose of reality: Hospitals like TIHH have proven that our all-digital environment can create an efficient and effective work environment. We've reduced costs and improved satisfaction for patients, doctors, and staff, all while improving the quality of care. But instead taking a hard look at their own operations, the larger not-for-profit hospital systems have realized that it's easier and less traumatic to work toward creating state and federal legislation. To this end, efforts are underway to attempt to create a permanent law or moratorium on the development, building, and growth of so-called "niche" hospitals, both at the federal and state levels, with Certificate of Need (CON) mandates. It's done with a Chicken Little, "the sky is falling" attitude that is meant to scare everyone into believing that competition from niche hospitals will drive the not-for-profit systems out of business, the end result being that patients will not be able to get care.

Nothing is further from the truth.

The reality is, competition has been proven to provide better results, services, products, and care in every industry in the world. Indeed, the Justice Department and the Federal Trade Commission recently issued a statement indicating that competition is good and should always be encouraged. Furthermore, the initial findings of MedPac (a Medicare cost agency) demonstrated that not-for-profits are showing better bottom lines in recent years due to increased competition, which has forced them to reevaluate how they provide care and services. Allowing competition to continue to work will result in improved costs and customer satisfaction over the next few years.

I'm not the only one who thinks specialty hospitals are the way of the future. Recently, and for the first time, the American Medical Association (AMA) House of Delegates passed an opinion letter that supports physician-owned specialty hospitals. This is the first time in memory that the AMA and the American Hospital Association have taken opposite positions on a topic. It just goes to show you that physicians are fed up with the current state of healthcare.

The Stark Laws

Most legislation on this issue to date has focused on the physician ownership of hospitals. In particular, the Stark laws essentially convey that doctors who invest in hospitals over utilize those hospitals and drive up healthcare costs. I will not debate the fact that there are some bad apples out there, hospitals whose ownership is driven solely as a profit model for physicians; you'll find similar problems in any industry. These are an extremely small minority when it comes to niche hospitals, however—perhaps 10 of the 100 or so specialty hospitals, out of the 5,000+ hospitals in the United States. This is a ridiculously low percentage.

For the remaining 90 or so specialty hospitals nationwide, the primary driver for physician ownership is not increased profitability for doctors. Rather, it's so that doctors can have a say in the care provided to their patients. The very reason specialty hospitals *exist* is because the CEOs for large, not-for-profit hospitals have yet to address the inefficient operations that cause physician frustration. Indeed, doctors' complaints about hospital operations fall on deaf ears. The result? Doctors at not-for-profit hospitals are left to grapple every day with poor care, poor accessibility, poor scheduling, dysfunctional silo-type operations, and competition for limited dollars.

Our future model for success *must* include the voice of physicians. If you truly want a successful operation, the physicians must be in control of the service line or hospital. And therein lies the problem. The not-for-profit world does not want to give up control. They would rather fight on the legislative front than give power to the very individuals who should and do have the greatest positive impact and influence on cost and quality.

David Veillette, FACHE

A Key Solution: Partnering with Not-for-Profits

One way to tackle the problem is for specialty hospitals to partner with not-for-profit systems. For example, we at TIHH are partnered with Community Health Network, a not-for-profit system. TIHH provides all the open-heart surgical services for the network, which eliminates duplication of services. In addition, TIHH purchases several millions of dollars of staff and services from our partner. Because we at TIHH have our own ER, we must by law accept all patients without regard or concern for payment, which eliminates any potential accusations of profit skimming. Our model is a win-win for TIHH and for our not-for-profit partner, helping to provide high-quality and low-cost care to all.

Using Legislation to Improve Healthcare

The legislation that not-for-profit hospitals are lobbying for, which would effectively enable them to retain a monopoly, would only further damage our already ailing system. That would be tragic for everyone. There is a way to use legislation to improve healthcare, however. First, I believe that a law could be designed to address the so-called "cherry picker" issue. If a specialty or physician-owned hospital can demonstrate three important elements, it would be in compliance:

- It must be aligned with a not-for-profit system. The redundancies and/or duplication of services must be eliminated and focused at one location.

- The governing board structure must be comprised with significant, if not majority, representation of physicians from the hospital's specialty area.

- The specialty hospital must provide an ER that is open 24 hours a day, seven days a week, 365 days a year. Arrangements can then be made with the partner system hospital for appropriate transfers back and forth of non-specialty patients. Here's an example of how this works. At TIHH, each patient who enters our ER is assessed. If the patient is "treatable and streetable," regardless of illness, care is provided at the TIHH ER. Likewise, if the patient's condition is deemed unstable or critical, regardless of illness, he or she is admitted and treated by TIHH. Once the patient has been treated and is stable, but requires further non-cardiac care, he or she is transferred to our sister hospital for appropriate care. The same process is used by our sister hospitals. When a cardiac patient arrives at one of their ERs, that patient is treated; when the patient is stable, however, he or she is transferred to our facility, regardless of the patient's ability to pay. This type of structure adds tremendous benefit for our not-for-profit partners, for TIHH, and most importantly, for our doctors and patients.

In addition, instead of looking at what is a perceived negative of niche and digital hospitals, allowing bad apples and self-serving, monopolistic organizations to prompt the creation of laws that will do more damage than good, legislation should be focused on requiring healthcare systems to bring their organizations into the future through the broad-based use of information technology. As I've demonstrated throughout this book, IT can enable any hospital—whether it's a general acute care organization or a specialty facility—to develop and implement an efficient model for operation.

David Veillette, FACHE

Regulatory Bodies

Beyond current legislative issues, we in healthcare face a host of inconsistencies and inefficiencies with regard to regulations and regulatory bodies. As but one example, consider the Joint Commission on Accreditation of Healthcare Organizations—JCAHO for short. JCAHO's mission, as stated on its Web site, is to "continuously improve the safety and quality of care provided to the public through the provision of healthcare accreditation and related services that support performance improvement in healthcare organizations." In order for a hospital to receive reimbursements from Medicare, Medicaid, and other types of insurance, it must be accredited by JCAHO or by a similar body. In my opinion, however, this regulatory body provides little benefit to hospitals or healthcare organizations. Specifically this body that is paid for by the Hospitals it surveys and if the purpose is to " ensure Quality" it is somewhat related to the "fox guarding the Hen House". How can an organization that is paid for by the certification they provide ensure an unbiased evaluation when their existence is dependant on finding issues and/or opportunities that require a need for a report. If JCAHO were funded by other sources that do not require the need to find fault then perhaps they would have some validity. Additionally this approach and evaluation provides a paper trial with enormous cost in staff and creates a punitive environment atmosphere. No one works well in a punitive state and this creates hospitals to not focus on quality but to merely prepare for the survey. This is similar to a teacher teaching the answers to a test in order to get a 100% pass rate. It actually defeats the original purpose of the objective.

In order to accredit a healthcare organization, JCAHO, among other things, conducts a survey visit. Prior to such a visit, it is incumbent upon the healthcare organization's staff to gather the required documentation and otherwise prepare. This process involves mountains of unnecessary paperwork, wasted man-hours, and cost. Not surprisingly, prior to a survey visit, morale is low, absenteeism is high, and the additional costs incurred are ludicrous. Worse, although this used to be an abuse that occurred every two to three years, now JCAHO can now spring a surprise visit on your organization any time after the first year of accreditation, making the process a year-round paranoia instead of a bi-annual headache. For what purpose? Has JCAHO accreditation resulted in a substantial improvement in healthcare quality? Hardly. To be fair to JCAHO, it is attempting to make changes but it's simply too little, too late.

Another example of a burdensome regulatory body is the Federal Drug Administration (FDA). Although I strongly believe the FDA provides benefits and has a responsibility to protect the public, I can't help but wonder, why does it take years to approve new drugs and devices? Why is the price tag for new technology in foreign countries one-third of what it is here in the U.S.? Why are pharmaceutical costs so much lower outside the U.S.? Why does Medicare not approve reimbursements for new technologies until FDA approval is received? And then, why do they often deny reimbursement for an additional year while waiting for an impact study? Pharmaceutical companies and device businesses market these products to doctors and patients, knowing that hospitals will not be able to recover these costs. So who pays for these drugs and devices? Sooner or later, we all do.

Hospitals are the victim in this whirlwind. Bureaucracy abounds. With their demand for paper trails and their looming threat of punitive authority, these regulatory bodies aren't serving anyone well. If I can use IT to improve my bottom line and ease the documentation nightmare, why can't they? In my view, they need to be totally redesigned into a logical and cooperative structure. They need to educate and assist healthcare organizations without demanding paper trails. Punitive authority needs to be removed.

The bottom line? The government, legislators, and regulatory bodies could have a positive impact on our current healthcare crisis or a significant negative impact. The choice will be theirs. I sincerely hope that these groups can separate the wheat from the chaff when listening to the rhetoric of not-for-profit organizations and self-serving certifying bodies. Most importantly, I hope they will allow those who can provide sensible answers to do so in an open and competitive environment.

Final Thoughts

"Even if you're on the right track, you'll get nowhere if you just sit there."

—Will Rogers

We are an industry—not to mention a nation—of complacent people, but we can't afford to stay that way. The status quo just doesn't work any longer. For this reason, I urge you to shake things up! Take the lead. Get involved. Walk around your facility. Talk to your people; together, you'll devise some brilliant solutions. Work with your Congressional representatives to ensure that your interests are served. Be fanatical about serving your customers. Finally, take the plunge with some changes. Yes, you'll have to open your mind and loosen the purse strings. Ask yourself: Are you going to jump on board, or are you going to be left behind? I believe most of us chose this profession to help people and to make a difference in the world. How are you measuring up?

Healthcare issues are global, yet profoundly personal. You are almost certain to experience a healthcare crisis – either personally or with a spouse, child, parent or friend. I can think of no other industry that has a more pervasive stronghold on our lives.

During my 35 years in healthcare, I've seen progress and backslides. I've seen miracles and devastation. Yet I remain optimistic. I continue to have a passion for this industry and all the people who work in it, and I have been honored to meet many of you during the course of my career. We make great strides every day! It's critical that we all work together and share our best practices. To this end, I invite your comments. Please contact me at CardconInc@insightbb.com. I look forward to hearing from you.

About the Author

David Veillette is President and Chief Executive Officer (CEO) of The Indiana Heart Hospital, the nation's first all digital specialty hospital. He was previously CEO of the Oklahoma Heart Center, LLC. He also is the President and CEO of Cardcon, Inc., a consulting firm that specializes in cardiovascular programs and services. He is a Fellow of the American College of Healthcare Executives.

Veillette received national recognition as the winner of the 2004 Louis Sullivan Award from the Workgroup for Electronic Data Interchange, which recognizes individuals who have distinguished themselves through their leadership, vision, and achievements in advancing the overall quality and efficiency of healthcare.

Veillette earned his bachelor's degree in chemistry, his master's degree in business, and his Ph.D. in management studies. He has more than 35 years experience in the cardiovascular field in both clinical and administrative leadership roles in many locations throughout the country. Veillette has earned national registry status in cardiovascular, perfusion, radiology, and pulmonary technologies. Starting his career as a scrub technician in a CATH lab in the late 1960s gave him the clinical experience to work closely with and understand the needs of physicians. He has had the privilege of working in both not-for-profit and for-profit healthcare environments. This experience managing multiple departments, in multiple environments, in many locations across the country has provided him with unique insight into many of the issues facing healthcare today. Veillette has consulted many organizations in developing and improving cardiovascular services. He is a constant lecturer, nationally and internationally, on the future model of healthcare and how to improve hospital efficiencies.

Over the years, Veillette has been the Chairman of the American Heart Association Heart Walk in both Oklahoma City and Indianapolis. He is a Paul Harris Fellow of Rotary International and is currently the Vice President of the Fishers Rotary in Fishers, Indiana.

If you would like to order additional copies of this book, please visit www.hospitalsincrisis.com.

If you would like information about group discounts or to schedule a speaking engagement with David Veillette, please call 317/845-9345.

You can also fax orders to: 317/251-2585.

Fax order:

Name: _____

Address: _____

City: _____ State: _____ Zip: _____

Phone: (_____) _____

_____ Visa/MasterCard

_____ American Express

Card Number: __ __ __ __ __ __ __ __ __ __ __ __ __ __

Exp. Date: ____ / ____

Daytime Telephone: (_____) _____

Please send _____ copies @ $19.95

Shipping:	Please add shipping & handling		
	First book:	$5.75	_____
	Each add'l book	3.38	_____

Sales tax (IN residents – add 5%) _____

Total: _____

Notes

Notes

Notes

Notes

Made in the USA
Lexington, KY
11 December 2009